Good Foods/Bad Foods
A Little Book of Common Sense Nutrition

Judith A. DeCava

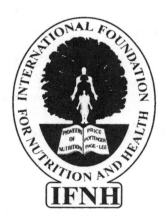

INTERNATIONAL FOUNDATION FOR NUTRITION AND HEALTH
SAN DIEGO, CA 92109

DeCava, Judith A., 1950-
Good Foods/Bad Foods
ISBN 978-0-984-0695-9-0

First published and dsitributed in 2009 by
International Foundation for Nutrition and Health
3963 Mission Blvd.
San Diego, CA 92109
Phone: (858-488-8932 • FAX: (858) 488-2566
www.ifnh.org •e-mail: ifnh@ifnh.org

Typesetting and design by Alternative Publishing

Cover design by Bluewater Designs

Printed in U.S.A.

CONTENTS

ACKNOWLEDGEMENTS

Heartfelt thanks to:

- All my clients throughout the years who gave me the best education I could ever receive.
- John Brady who initiated and managed this project as well as made suggestions to make it meaningful and fun.
- Jeff Archer for his editing expertise and help beyond the call of duty.
- David Tannen who occasionally tosses me a juicy tidbit of information that stirs me to write.
- Mike who never ceases to believe in me.

— Judy DeCava

INTRODUCTION

Good Foods/Bad Foods, what a title. We all remember when our mothers badgered us to eat all the food on our plate, telling us "There are children in China who are starving," pushing the notion that macaroni with Velveeta cheese was good for us.

My mother, like most mothers of her day, thought if the product was advertised on television and radio, it had to be safe and healthy. Unfortunately, we are discovering that isn't always the case. Good foods, in most cases, are organically-raised and often found at your local farmers market. They are therapeutic and full of vitamins and minerals. Bad foods, refined and devitalized, such as white flour and sugar, are not only bad for us; they are dangerous to our overall health

Today, the nation seems to be deeply divided over what to do about healthcare. With all the proposals I have not heard one word about prevention with the emphasis on staying healthy. The pioneers of nutrition like Doctors Royal Lee, Weston Price, Francis Pottenger, Melvin Page, and the first head of the FDA, Dr. Harvey Wiley, found themselves fighting for their professional lives because of their outspoken beliefs regarding the therapeutic value of whole natural foods. They felt our government needed to recognize that eating healthy food was the first step in having a hearty vibrant population.

Dr. Wiley impounded several trainloads of white flour and designated the product as a toxic substance. As a result, he was forced to retire from his position in the government. The flour mills quickly formed an alliance with the pharmaceutical companies and added synthetic vitamins to white flour, giving the impression the public was protected. Then, both interests contributed heavily to the senators and congressmen who would endorse their agenda. Today, it seems we are faced with the same dilemma that Dr. Wiley and Dr. Lee endured.

For example, I read about a doctor in Panama City, Florida, Dr. Jason Newsom, who was fired from his position as head of the Bay County Health Department for trying to make people aware of the dangers of unhealthy food. The focus of his campaign was on the dangers to our health from fast foods, white flour and white sugar, with a special emphasis on donuts. He even had the audacity to ban donuts, fast food and soft drinks from the office.

He then posted slogans like "Hamburger Spare Tire," "French Fries Thunder Thighs," and, worst of all, he parodied "America Runs on Dunkin'," the Dunkin' Donuts' corporate slogan, with, "America Dies on Dunkin'," to promote his campaign for a healthier diet and lifestyle.

That was too much for this Gulf Coast tourist town where 39 percent of all adults were overweight in 2007 and one in four was considered obese.

Two prominent lawyers, who owned Dunkin' Donuts franchises, opposed the doctor's campaign. They went to one of the County commissioners, who also owned a donut shop, and. this new opposition was a enough of an influencing factor in swaying the tide against the health advocate. Does this mean health is a consideration only if it's convenient? If so, at what cost? Unfortunately, it costs us all through skyrocketing healthcare costs.

Sixty two percent of U.S. citizens are overweight with 31% considered obese, compared to 3.2% of Japanese and Koreans. Childhood obesity in the United States has more than tripled in the past two decades. According to a 2007 report, the U.S. Surgeon General stated that obesity is responsible for 300,000 deaths every year. The National Institutes of Health proclaimed that an estimated 850,000 to 1.7 million Americans have type 1 diabetes. Of those, about 125,000 are kids 19 and under. An additional 30,000 Americans develop type 1 diabetes every year, 13,000 of whom are children. Another estimated 16 million Americans are suffering from type 2 diabetes.

What's a good alternative? Go to the farmer's market, look around and notice the beautiful colors of the rainbow in all the fruit and vegetable stands. This kaleidoscope of colors represents nature's benefit to our health. For an example, anthocyanins make blueberries blue and can help to keep your mind sharp and focused. Tomatoes get their color from lycopene, which is said to help prevent prostate cancer.

The next time you go shopping look at those wonderful colors in a different way. When you see the green color of broccoli, green cabbage and kale, remember these cruciferous vegetables provide compounds called indoles and isothiocyanates, which may help prevent cancer by increasing the production of enzymes that can help remove toxins from the body.

Look at the corn, summer squash, wax beans, green beans, arugula, chard, collards, lettuce, artichokes and mustard greens. Many of the yellow and green vegetables are excellent sources of lutein and zeaxanthin: phytochemicals which accumulate in the eyes and help prevent age-related macular degeneration, a major cause of blindness in older people. Leafy greens are also rich in beta carotene..

Orange-colored produce, such as oranges, papaya, apricots, cantaloupe, carrots, mango, and tangerines, all contain alpha and beta carotene. The body converts these compounds into the active form of vitamin A, which helps keep your eyes, bones and immune system healthy and strong. These phytochemicals also operate as antioxidants, clearing away disease-promoting free radicals.

Lastly, the deep reds, blues and purples of fruits or vegetables show they are full of anthocyanins, antioxidants associated with keeping the heart healthy and the brain functioning optimally. Do yourself a favor and round out your shopping list by choosing at least one of these fruits or vegetables: raspberries, strawberries, radishes, blackberries, blueberries and eggplant.

As I wander through the farmers market on my weekly trek, I can't help but find myself energized by the vibrant colors that are depicted on the cover of this book. Knowing the differences in real natural whole foods versus synthetic man-made or genetically-engineered products that are dramatically described within the pages of this book is a subject that I have been pursuing for years. It is from the therapeutic properties of real food that health can be enjoyed and maintained. Why this simple truth is so hard to convince the mainstream public is a quandary for me and others who work in the field of nutrition. But, it is a challenge that we readily accept.

Judy DeCava does not waste our time with the standard look at a topic. She doesn't hype you up on how you can lose 30 pounds in 15 days or how to cure all diseases with this secret herb just discovered in the Amazon rain forests. Instead she's designed each chapter as a steppingstone on your path to health by filling it with information backed by thoroughly and accurately-cited research. Many books on nutrition are lean on supplying sources of information, making the merit of the entire work somewhat dubious. But, after all the explaining of her research (earlier and current), she adds a delightful section called "Food For Thought." In this, she supplies us with quotes and information from experts in the field. Each portion has commentary that either supports or denies the mainstream thought that DeCava highlighted in the chapter. This is a refreshing concept for those who want to learn facts, not merely one person's opinion.

This book will take you on a journey of truth and reality that can be sobering yet exciting. She exposes the silver-tongued Madison Avenue media manager's half-truths that many of our politicians seem to have turned a blind eye to. This makes one realize how corporate greed has led us down a road that seems to have lost any moral accountability. This situation is ours to change. Armed with more knowledge, we can make a difference in our own health and the health of those around us.

The Greek philosopher *Heraclitus* once said, "Education is to light a fire, not fill a bucket." Enjoy the journey, remember life is good.

John R Brady
International Foundation for Nutrition and Health

Good Foods/Bad Foods

Chapter One

What's the Problem?

You are being cheated. It's not that you're just being cheated of money, but you're being cheated of health and probably years of your life. The problem is what we are eating. We've been led to believe that the food we buy will not hurt us and that it will supply us with the nourishment we need to be well. Instead, we're eating items that are far from what Nature intended we consume. Things we put into our mouths are industrialized, commercialized, diminished in nourishment, and toxic in many cases. The result is that many of us are suffering from *malnutrition*. What? In a country with more food than any other country? With more than two-thirds of North Americans overweight? Yes. Malnutrition means you don't consume enough needed nutrients *or* you consume too many calories that are deficient in needed nutrients. You can eat plenty of food and still be undernourished. In fact, you can eat too much food and be undernourished.

I was struck by a headline in the "letters to the editor" section of the prominent medical journal, *The Lancet*, that stated: "Malnutrition Kills Directly, not Indirectly." Malnutrition is a direct, straightforward cause—not just an underlying, indirect cause—of failing health, disease and death. You and I may not die tomorrow from malnutrition. But we can be promoting a long, slow descent into illness, disease, and our own demise. According to one review, an estimated 50% of people have a chronic (long-standing) physical condition needing some form of medical treatment. About 35% of young adults have at least one chronic condition and far more chronic illnesses occur in older adults.

Cheer up—there is good news. This situation can change for you personally.

Each of us can get back on track so that our own food system is in sync with our body's needs. We can reclaim our understanding of what real, healthy food is. We can add nutritional supplements to make up for some of the deficits we have developed. Many of us are already trying to do that. But there are many conflicting and confusing claims and recommendations. So we may need some guidance. I'm hoping I can be one of your guides and I'll back up the information I offer with science and my own experience as well as the experience of many other health professionals.

Here's the story. Most North Americans don't eat a healthy, nutritious diet. They don't realize that they're eating lots of things that don't qualify as real food. I think most people already know or suspect this. An FDA (Food and Drug Administration) survey found that 90% of Americans say they're actively trying to eat a healthy diet. But there is only "mixed adherence" to their goals. Only 70% of women and 54% of men thought that nutrition was important to take into account when food shopping. Young adults, aged 18 to 34, were the least likely to consider nutrition very important or to avoid unhealthy food choices. Since you picked up this book to read, you are obviously one in the minority who is willing to take nutrition into account, who wants to actively do something about it. Good for you (literally).

Most people don't always know the difference between real foods and nonfoods. So they eat what tastes good to them (often, what they are used to eating). Or they eat what advertising attracts them to, or what is convenient or handy. And, unfortunately, most of us have lost touch with our natural body indicators—we don't know what our bodies are trying to tell us. Each one of us needs to learn to listen to our body; in this way we can be happily surprised at the wisdom it imparts.

We've been led astray. The "food" industry—or, as I call it, the "nonfood" industry—doesn't want to be associated with poor health and growing girths, so it offers low-fat, non-fat, low-carb, reduced sugar, low-sodium, cholesterol-free, low-calorie, negative-calorie, herb-boosted, 'enriched,' artificially-fortified everything. It throws in a little bit of whole grain (with chemical preservatives), fruits or vegetables (in amounts you need a microscope to find and processed so much they have to be artificially colored or flavored), flaxseed (often rancid or over-cooked), or some other healthful-sounding ingredient(s). Potato chips with no trans fats, soy-boosted low-carb pizza, and chocolate bars containing no sugar all sound good, but these nonfoods are still nonfoods. Often one unhealthy industrialized ingredient is substituted for another, and sometimes new ingredients are worse than old ingredients. Advertisements boast about the nutrient-contents of products that contain manufactured chemicals that imitate nutrient parts. Folks, we are in sad shape if we believe any of this can make up for not eating real food. But the promotions by the food industry are pervasive and sound convincing.

Of course, the FDA doesn't entirely help the situation. It does allow health claims to be made on, shall we say, questionable food products. One recent example is the FDA's approval for a qualified health claim that allows manufacturers to state, "Very limited and preliminary scientific evidence suggests that eating about one tablespoon (16 grams) of corn oil daily may reduce the risk of heart disease because of the unsaturated fat content in corn oil." Although the claim acknowledges only weak scientific evidence supports such a claim, it doesn't reveal that the evidence is pitifully weak and that the claim may be more than wrong—it may be misleading. Corn oil, virtually always refined (which includes high heat that transforms the fatty acids into more toxic versions) is also high in omega-6 fatty acids and virtually void of omega-3 fatty acids. Most North Americans are deficient in omega-3s, and getting a lot more omega-6s can worsen that problem. Cooking with corn oil will lead to the formation of heart and blood-vessel-damaging lipid peroxides. So using more corn oil won't help. There is far more evidence that it may promote the development of heart disease. But you won't see that on a bottle of corn oil.

Some dieticians and doctors will tell you that all foods (real foods and nonfoods) can fit into a balanced diet. But, come on, some foods *are* certainly much better than others. Some of us have figured that out. Some have not. If you're trying to eat healthier real foods, you can consider yourself a trendsetter, motivated to stay healthy and filled with vitality. Making healthier food choices may require a little extra effort and willpower, but it's not only worth it; it makes eating more enjoyable. According to the results of a 2008 study, most Americans are not consuming the most nutrient-dense forms of foods. Instead, the majority are eating too many nonfoods.

According to a University of California analysis of a national survey, one-third or *more* of the typical American diet consists of outrageously blatant *nonfoods*—items that don't even fit into any of the food groups (dairy, fruit, grains, meat and beans, and vegetables). The remaining two-thirds or *less* of the diet is supposed to supply *all* (100% of) the nutrients and other components needed to obtain or maintain some semblance of health. Yet these remaining foods that are supposed to give you everything you need are often raised or processed in ways that lower their nutritional value or place stress on the body. Many of them are nonfoods too. Therefore, most Americans are eating very little if any real food. Nonfoods certainly mess things up, such as causing the body to lose nutrients and giving it alien and toxic substances to deal with. The end result is unhealthy, hungry bodies—people are starving for what their bodies need.

So what do they do? Since their bodies are hungry, they eat more. Americans are eating, on average, 140 more pounds of food each year than they did a decade ago. Their bodies are hungry because nonfoods don't supply the nutrient value needed. They don't eat enough real food with real nutrients. Most folks in the US are suffering from an excess of empty calories and a deficiency of nutrients. People are eating *more* of what they *don't* need (nonfood) because their bodies are hungry for what they *do* need (sufficient nourishment from real food).

Although many people try to approach this intelligently, the food industry lures them along a perverse path. So they eat nonfoods that are enriched or fortified with so-called "nutrients." And they take supplements. Two-thirds of Americans take supplements to prevent disease, increase energy, enhance their appearance, lose weight, reduce stress, and improve fitness. Supplements are supposed to justify or make up for all the nonfood eaten and all the real food not eaten. This may certainly appear to make sense, yet there are things that people don't know and aren't taught. For one thing, the "nutrients" used to enrich or fortify products, and most all of the supplements on the market are chemicals taken from substances that are not foods, separated from foods, or (most-likely) manufactured in a laboratory. They are not foods. They don't even come close. So they won't work like real foods and they can cause problems as well. Many scientific studies are showing this. Foods "work" in preventing or helping various health conditions and diseases. Then when scientists isolate a specific, single nutrient in a food—what they believe to be the "active ingredient—and give it to people, it doesn't "work."

Thus, a lot of recent research has wound up showing that manufactured chemical- or isolated-nutrient supplements don't combat the wide range of health problems as was hoped. For example, a separated part of vitamin E (as used in most supplements) does not prevent cardiovascular disease, though foods containing vitamin E complex do. Beta-carotene supplements—fabricated in a factory—don't reduce the risk of lung cancer like foods containing carotenes and other cooperative coworkers. Folate (folic acid) supplementation was thought to help prevent heart disease since foods rich in this nutrient definitely appear to; they didn't work. Many other examples could be offered, but you get the point.

People keep getting sick. What's the next step they take? Very often, drugs. Just over half (51%) of *insured* Americans take drugs for chronic conditions—conditions that, for the most part, could be avoided by good food and a healthy lifestyle. Among insured people aged 45 to 65, 70% of women and 60% of men take drugs for chronic conditions. The numbers for people over 65 are 81% for women and 74% for men.

More than half of the folks over 65 take three or more such drugs; about one-fifth of them take five or more. More than one in five people take drugs for high blood pressure; one in seven take cholesterol-lowering drugs. More young adults are taking prescribed drugs too. Almost half of women and one-third of men aged 20 to 44 take drugs for chronic conditions; their leading drugs are antidepressants.

Side effects of drugs are now the fourth leading cause of death in this country (following heart disease, cancer, and stroke). The *Journal of the American Medical Association* published findings that showed adverse drug reactions caused 1.4 million emergency room visits in 2004 and 2005. Medications taken as prescribed are estimated to kill some 100,000 Americans a year. This is considered to be a conservative estimate; another study figured that this number should be doubled. According to a survey reported in the *Joint Commission Journal on Quality and Patient Safety*, 4.3 million North Americans went to their doctors in 2001 for drug side effects (or, in medical terms, "adverse drug reactions"). Furthermore, the number of adverse reactions and fatalities attributable to prescription drugs is actually many times the number actually reported. Drugs are advertised on television to urge consumers to demand them from their doctors. The Internet allows doctors to prescribe drugs without seeing patients or learning their case histories. This can only increase the grim statistics.

It's not that drugs are always bad. Sometimes they are necessary and perhaps even life-saving. It's the misuse and over-use of drugs that create huge problems. According to the Centers for Disease Control, prescription drug use has risen from approximately 4 drugs per person in 1995-1996 to 5.2 drugs in 2001-2002. Almost half of all US adults take at least one prescription drug, and half of older persons take three or more. Sickness and disease are not drug deficiencies. Have you ever wondered why a health problem is called a "medical condition" that "your doctor can treat?" A problem becomes a "medical condition" when a drug has been manufactured to treat the symptoms. That's why "restless leg syndrome" (or RLS) is now a medical condition—a drug company has a new drug for the symptoms. (RLS is common in people with low iron levels or nerve-related problems—why not eliminate toxins that can worsen it and supplement with foods and nutrients that support iron metabolism and nerve health, such as calcium, magnesium, potassium, and the vitamin B complex?) Remember, all drugs are toxic, many are outright poisons. They should be used very carefully and judiciously. Also remember that drugs do not heal. Drugs are not what make people healthy. They may alleviate—mask—symptoms but they don't get to the underlying cause(s) in most cases.

Aspirin, for example, may ease a headache, but it doesn't help the cause of the headache. This brings to mind the wife of a client of mine. The client was distressed because his wife's doctor said she could take several aspirin each day to cope with her headaches. She could not be dissuaded from this course. One day, the client came home to find his wife dead on their living room floor. She had an aneurysm, an abnormal "bubble" on a blood vessel in her head. It had leaked a little, something that may have been stopped if her blood clotted properly. But, because of the continuous diet of aspirin, she hemorrhaged and bled to death. (Many people take aspirin each day to prevent a heart attack or stroke, but then find they bruise much too easily, or their gums bleed, or they bleed excessively from a small cut, or they start experiencing irritation in their stomachs that may lead to bleeding ulcers.)

Various other examples come to mind such as the understandably distressed (freaked out) man in his 50s who became impotent due to the blood pressure medication his doctor prescribed. The doctor agreed to take him off the drug and, with healthy dietary changes, some weight loss, and supplementation with food concentrates, the blood pressure came down and, shall we say, his spirits came up. Then there was the menopausal woman who was given an antidepressant, only to develop a tremor. This terrified her since her father died with Parkinson's disease—she thought she was developing the same. After quitting the drug, the tremors stopped, and with some support from diet, exercise, and food (and herb) supplements, she breezed through menopause. A three-year-old boy developed kidney problems after being given a certain antibiotic prescribed by a pediatrician over the phone. It took almost two years of good nutrition to totally regain healthy kidney function.

Many doctors realize the problem with drugs, don't want to be merely drug peddlers, and seek other, safer, gentler, more natural therapies. For example, they use supplements and herbs. However, there is a danger that supplements are viewed and used simply as safer drugs. There is a tremendous difference between drugs and drug effects versus real foods and nutritional effects. But the difference may be blurred in the minds of many people. Scientists can confuse them.

The usual concept of science suggests that an analysis of the parts of something is sufficient to understand the whole. Unfortunately, this doesn't work with real people and real food. They are much too complicated, there are individual differences, there is a natural synergy (all parts affect all other parts), and taking foods apart destroys their ability to function. Humans and foods are living, animated. Dissect their parts and you lose the life force, the interactions, the interconnections, the ecology—the symbiosis. To put it mildly, something gets lost. No wonder that scientists are learning that the relationship of foods and diet to health is "complex, not easily broken down into component parts," as *Tufts University Health & Nutrition Letter* puts it.

Unfortunately, when scientists study nutrients, they don't usually use whole real foods. They use a nutrient part, often manufactured artificially. But just as your heart will not pump very long after removing it from your body, so too, an isolated nutrient can't perform as a functional nutrient once separated from its whole food complex. Neither can it act as the whole complex. The sum of the parts does not equal the whole.

Another problem with the scientific method is measurement. How can a separated part or chemical imitation of a separated part of a nutrient network be measured based on its actions outside the body (in Petri dishes or test tubes) or inside the body when it is something the body does not recognize as "food?" This would be like judging the ability of a whole football team when there is only one player on the field. Even if the player was the quarterback—an important member—little can be surmised without the help of the rest of the team. Worse yet, suppose the player was not a real member of the team—just looked like it because he wore the uniform. Or suppose most of the team does show up—except the quarterback. What you would have is chaos, lack of organization, so that nothing much could be accomplished.

So too with nutrients. Taking out of a food what is assumed to be an important part destroys the team. Imitating a part—making a synthetic look-alike—is even worse. Single factors separated or synthesized are *not* real nutrients anymore than one team member or a counterfeit team member is the whole team. If only one part is missing, the team cannot accomplish its goal effectively. The team is not functional. Neither is the nutrient. They are both phonies. What you create is biochemical chaos.

Furthermore, an important point was made by Michael Pollan, author of *In Defense of Food*. He says that the ideology of nutritionism is actually harmful to us. Nutritionism is a belief that foods are simply a collection of nutrients and that we need "experts" who "design our foods (and supplements) and tell us how to eat." One of the problems with this is the focus scientists usually give to one nutrient at a time while they ignore the effects of processing foods as well as the combination of nutrients within a single food and in the total diet. We don't know or understand all the components of real foods. We don't know or understand everything the body does with these components or the individual variations or the effects of an entire lifestyle. Nutritionism looks at food only as a means to supply fuel and to advance physical health. But food is much more complicated and intricate and plays many more roles.

Another complication: You are unique. Each one of us is unique. It's called biochemical individuality. This means we all have our own individual needs, individual abilities to handle and process different chemicals and chemical combinations, individual responses and reactions, even individual levels of nutritional stores and other natural biochemicals. How can scientists measure this uniqueness? How can they determine exactly what amount of specific nutrients you need? They can't. Saying there is a minimum requirement or optimal dosage is thus meaningless. It's different with real foods. You have the ability to absorb more of less of any nutrient network in real foods, depending on your needs and circumstances at that particular time. This is called selective absorption.

Your nutritional needs change. Children are different from young adults. Adults are different from older adults. Your circumstances change. Your body changes. When you have a health issue, your needs are different or more or less than when you don't have that health issue. Pregnancy, nursing, menopause, and other hormonal adjustments mean your body's needs change. The amount of physical work or exercise you do, the amount and type of stress you're under—and how you react to it—the amount and quality of sleep you get, and so many other things affect your nutritional requirements. Real whole foods give your body the discretion to take what it needs in the amounts it needs as long as we are consuming the foods that contain those requirements.

If a scientific study uses a manufactured imitation of a nutrient part, the results can be different from those of a study that uses a separated part taken from a food. If a study looks at whole foods, results can be very different from either of these. If a fake imitation or separated part is used at a certain dosage, say 50 milligrams of vitamin B_1 (thiamin), people would have various reactions depending on their unique ability to process, recombine, and get rid of the chemical. If animals were used, results could be very unlike those from humans. No wonder reports on scientific studies are contradictory, confusing, and sometimes downright dumbfounding.

In Nature, the amounts of various components of real foods and whole herbs will vary. It's not so much the quantity of a single ingredient that matters as much as the quality— the synergy, the interaction of all the components—that make a food or herb "work." Separated and imitation "nutrients" may "prove" to cause certain reactions in one set of experiments only to be disproved in others. Some synthetic imitations even appear to worsen conditions rather than help.

This brings to mind a woman, Evelyn, who contacted me in desperation after consulting several doctors about her stubborn, long-lasting case of hives. She couldn't even rest or sleep because of her constantly sore and itchy skin. None of the doctors picked up on the fact that she was taking large amounts of ascorbic acid—a synthetic part of the vitamin C complex. Ascorbic acid can cause hives. After stopping the ascorbic acid, getting the whole vitamin C complex in foods and supplements, and some extra support with green leafy vegetables and supplements containing them, the hives were gone. Evelyn was convinced that a miracle had occurred.

Scientists often try to apply drug rules to nutrients. Most supplements on the market—vitamins, minerals, amino acids, phytochemicals, fatty acids, herbs, and others—are designed, manufactured, and used in a drug-like manner. That's why many people look to supplements as "safe drugs." But drugs modify bodily functions. They stimulate or suppress to relieve a symptom or control a condition. They interfere with the normal processes of the body. A glance at the list of possible side effects of a drug makes this clear. A real nutrient is a substance that nourishes or feeds the body's cells and tissues.

When a body is ill, a drug compels the body to change something and keeps it under "control." Nutrients provide fuel the body can use to operate, repair, renew, and heal. Drugs—and drug-like supplements—jolt the body. They don't feed it. Only real foods feed the body and allow it to use the nutrients as it knows best. Drugs mean someone else is in control. Foods mean your body is in control.

Who or what is trusted the most for nutrition information? About 30% do not trust *any* source; 20% trust their doctors (the vast majority of whom get no education in nutrition); 13% trust the Internet. Americans are skeptics—no doubt because they are confused and concerned about all the contradictory and commercialized information they are 'fed' about nutrition. What about you?

(Data from Food Marketing Institute 2005)

Where Do North Americans Get Their Nutrition Information?

Source	
Magazines	46%
Internet	46%
Television	38%
Doctor	35%
Newspaper	34%
Friends and Family	33%
Books	30%
Grocery store	27%
Nutritionist and dietician	13%
Radio	13%
Pharmacist	7%

References:

Bachman, J.L., J. Reedy, et al, "Sources of Food Group Intakes Among the US Population," *Journal of the American Dietetic Association*, 2008: 108:804-14.

British Medical Journal, 2004: 329:369, cited in *What Doctors Don't Tell You*, Aug. 2008: 19(5):6-10.

Classen, D.C., S.L. Pestotnik, et al, "Adverse Drug Events in Hospitalized patients: Excess Length of Stay, Extra Costs, and Attributable Mortality," *Journal of the American Medical Association*, 1997: 277:301-306.

"Did you know...", *Health & Healing* Oct. 2002: 12(10):5.

Gaby, Alan R., "The Mainstreaming of Misinformation," *Townsend Letter*, Aug./Sept. 2007: 289/290:63.

Goldberg, B., "The Science of Deceit," *The John R Lee, MD, Medical Letter*, Apr. 2002:5.

Goldner, D., *Infinite Grace*, Charlottesville, NC: Hampton Roads Publishing Company, Inc., 1999.

"Good Intentions Lost on the Way to Grocery Store," *Tufts University Health & Nutrition Letter*, July 2008: 26(5):3.

Habicht, Jean-Pierre, "Malnutrition Kills Directly, not Indirectly," *The Lancet*, 24 May 2008: 371(9626):1749-50.

Hampton, Tracy, "Flawed Prescribing Practices Revealed," *Journal of the American Medical Association*, 8 Nov. 2006, 296(18):2191-2192.

"Healthy Foods in Fashion," *Tufts University Health & Nutrition Letter*, Apr. 2008: 26(2):3.

"If We Got Report Cards for Food Choices, There'd Be a Lot of Fs," *Tufts University Health & Nutrition Letter*, August 2004: 22(6):2 and "Junk Food, or Junky Food Choices?," Sept. 2003: 21(7):3.

Journal of the American Dietetic Association, 2008: 108:804-14.

"Junk Food," *Nutrition Week*, 29 Sept. 2000: 30(37):7, citing *American Journal of Clinical Nutrition*, Oct. 2000: 72(4):929-936.

Klotter, Jule, "Nutritionism," *Townsend Letter*, July 2008: 300:40, citing interview with Michael Pollan.

Kratz, A.M., "Pharmaceutical Compounding of Natural Products," *Townsend Letter for Doctors & Patients*, Oct. 2000: Is.207:126-127.

Lazarou, J., et al, "Incidence of Adverse Drug Reactions in Hospitalized Patients," *Journal of the American Medical Association*, 1998: 279(15):1200-1205.

Lee, Royal, "Skullduggery and Semantic Juggling in Food and Drug laws," lecture to meeting of the Lee Foundation, Spring 1955: *Lectures of Dr Royal Lee*, Vol.1, Fort Collins, CO: Selene River Press, 1998:189-192.

"Matters of Opinion & Taste," *Eating Well*, Fall 2004: 3(2):6, quoting Professor Gladys Block, UC Berkeley.

"Medication Nation," *UC Berkeley Wellness Letter*, Sept. 2008: 24(12):8.

Merck Manual, 17th Edition, Rahway, NJ: Merck Research Laboratories, 1997.

Ridder, Denise de, Rinie Geenen, et al, "Psychological Adjustment to Chronic Disease," *The Lancet*, 19 July 2008: 372(9634):246-255.

"Safety Concerns Grow Along with Dietary Supplement Use," *Nutrition Week*, Jan. 2002: 32(2):7.

Vastag, B., "Health Agencies Update," *Journal of the American Medical Association*, 2002: 288(11): 1342.

Wolfe, Sidney M., "Adverse Drug Reactions Cause 1.4 Million Emergency Room Visits in 2004 and 2005," *Worst Pills, Best Pills News*, Jan. 2007: 13(1):1-2, citing the *Journal of the American Medical Association*, 18 Oct. 2006.

Zhan, C., I. Arispe, et al, "Ambulatory Care Visits for Treating Adverse Drug Effects in the United States, 1995-2001," *Joint Commission Journal on Quality Patient Safety*, 2005: 31(7):372-8.

"25 years of Health & Nutrition Breakthroughs," *Tufts University Health & Nutrition Letter* March 2008: 26(1):4-5.

FOOD FOR THOUGHT

Nearly 80% of North Americans say they scrutinize nutrition labels of foods. Yet, even when the label lists unhealthy ingredients, 44% of people admit to buying the item anyway. Women place more importance on nutrition content than men do, and are more likely to check Nutrition Facts labels. Married men (maybe because they are influenced by their wives) are more likely to check labels than unmarried men. Younger people, ages 18 to 29, check for calories first. Then they're more likely to ignore any bad news on the nutrition label and buy unhealthy foods anyway—60% admit to ignoring labels even after reading them.

Reference: "A Feast for the Eyes," *Tufts University Health & Nutrition Letter,* Sept: 2006, 24(7):3.

It is estimated that more than $24 billion in national health care costs could be saved through the targeted use of nutritional supplements. Only five supplements were examined—calcium, folic acid, omega-3 fatty acids, glucosamine, and saw palmetto. Imagine what could be saved—in illness and disease as well as in dollars—if other nutritional supplements and good healthful foods were used.

Reference: DaVanzo, J., et al, "Improving Public Health, Reducing Health Care Costs: An Evidence-Based Study of Five Dietary Supplements," The Lewin Group, 22 Sept. 2004.

After flour is refined, it still tends to keep a yellowish tint which is not considered appealing. The yellow tint is removed by bleaching the flour, destroying any vestiges of vitamin E left after refining. The bleaching is done with chlorine dioxide gas. Better flours are naturally aged, allowing the air to bleach them. If you must use refined flour, get unbleached.

Ever wonder why you can't seem to duplicate the lightness and tenderness of commercial cakes? The reason is that they use chlorinated flour and special fat emulsifiers. To make the chlorinated flour, bleaching agents are mixed with chlorine gas.

WHAT'S THE PROBLEM?

Reference: Bader, Myles H., *2001 Food Secrets Revealed*, Las Vegas, NV: Northstar Publishing, 1997:14.

Recently the blood and urine of 13 people in Maine were analyzed. The presence of 46 dangerous chemicals were found—including arsenic, mercury, lead, PFCs (from Teflon, various cookware, and clothing), PBDEs (flame retardants, mostly found in fabrics), and phthalates (from plastics and cosmetics). Even tiny amounts of such chemicals are life-threatening since many of them degrade slowly building up in our bodies to higher and higher levels due to constant exposure and consumption. Babies and children are particularly susceptible. This kind of information always makes my blood boil!
Reference: *Acres USA*, "Toxic Humans," September 2007, 37(9):65.

Award-winning journalist Shannon Brownlee did her homework and wrote a book entitled *Overtreated: Why Too Much Medicine Is Making US Sicker and Poorer*. She insists that a whooping one-third of the health care you receive is unnecessary and potentially dangerous. I would add that a lot of health care could be avoided if we participated in more self-care—good food, regular exercise, simpler life-style—you know, the stuff we keep hearing about but don't always do.
Reference: "Diagnosis: Too Much Medicine?," *Health*, Sept. 2007: 21(7):94.

Chapter Two

WHAT HAPPENED TO OUR FOOD?

I guess I'd have to say that the food industry—commercialism of what we eat—happened to food. Most of the things that people eat are meant to be sold, not to be eaten. And I'm not alone in my viewpoint.

Many people in the nutrition and farming fields feel the same. For instance, Lola O'Rourke, a registered dietician and spokesperson for the American Dietetics Association, articulated what many others have stated: "People need to keep in mind that the food marketing machine exists for profits, not health. So it's important to look at the ingredients on the packages when you buy processed foods—and to try and use whole foods more."

What happened?

For one thing, modern farming/ranching methods. Huge agribusinesses have taken over where small family farms once existed. Production is astronomical but quality has plummeted. North Americans are probably the most well-fed, undernourished people in history. The soil has been depleted of natural nutrients and essential microorganisms and it is saturated with chemical fertilizers and pesticides. The soil can only give to plants what it has, so our foods contain far lower amounts of nutrients than they did 55 or 65 years ago. And, they contain far more poisonous residues.

Fruits and vegetables grown in the US in the 1990s had lower nutrient contents than those grown in the 1950s; anywhere from 6% to 76% less. Today's crops have up to 37% lower levels of nutrients than those grown in 1975. Animals used for food are deficient as well because they receive fewer nutrients in their feeds.

Dr. Firman E. Bear of Rutgers University looked at the mineral content of tomatoes, snap beans, cabbage, spinach and lettuce. Let's look at the tomato findings. Tomatoes from 67 farms in 10 different states had various mineral contents: the highest amount of manganese had 68 ppm (parts per million) while the lowest had 1 ppm. The average was a mere 4 ppm. The highest amount of copper he found was 53 ppm and the lowest was zero. The average was just 18.1 ppm of copper. Dr. Bear found that the average amounts were much closer to the lowest amounts in all the six minerals he tested. He provided evidence that the mineral contents of our food depend upon the mineral content of the soil where the food grew. Here's the kicker: Dr. Bear finished his study in 1948. Add 60 years of industrialized farming, the disappearance of minerals from our soils, and the nutrient scarcity in the plants grown in those soils, as well as the animals eating those plants, and you end up with major deficiencies in people eating those foods.

Artificial chemical fertilizers don't replenish the soil, they deplete it and create unbalance. Crops come from deficient soils because the chemicals in the fertilizers replace real nutrients in the plants when plant tissues are formed. For example, ammonium nitrate (the key compound in modern "fixed" nitrogen fertilizers) largely replaces nutrients like calcium, magnesium, and potassium in making plant tissue. When there is a lot of nitrogen from chemical fertilizers, plants increase protein production and decrease carbohydrate production. Isn't this a good thing? No. When the normal protein requirements of the plant have been met, the extra protein produced is in a storage form that contains lower amounts of essential amino acids. It's a poor quality protein—junk protein. Gluten in wheat is one example of a storage protein. Since the quality is poor and there's a lot more than normal, I have to attribute, at least in part, the growing incidence of gluten sensitivity (intolerance to wheat, rye, and barley) to this aberrant protein caused by synthetic fertilizers.

If not diluted, inorganic chemical fertilizers are faster-acting than organic fertilizers and can burn plants. They leach quicker from the soil and topsoil is used up. Loss of topsoil is a major problem. The plants may look okay, but they're not healthy. Pests and disease greatly threaten unhealthy crops, so pesticides are then applied. Weeds infiltrate in an attempt to rebalance the soil, so herbicides are applied. Mircroorganisms in the soil are destroyed and the soil eventually dies. Dead soil does not produce healthful food.

Have you ever actually seen an agribusiness in the works? I have: up close and personal. When I was in the Midwest, the area in which I lived and worked was surrounded by huge tracts of farm fields. In the early spring, small planes emitted a huge, awful-smelling cloud of herbicides over the fields. Within days, not one plant in those fields was alive. Anything living in the soil that was necessary for healthy plants, such as worms, microorganisms, and fungi, was also dead. Then came the chemically-treated seeds, followed routinely by more sprayings of pesticides. I developed multiple chemical and food sensitivities. My little dog developed tumors. I became extremely interested in what is now called environmental medicine.

Not only are we getting what we *don't* want—toxic residues—but we're *not* getting what we *do* want—healthful, nutritious foods. Back in 1924, Jack Gaerity, author of *Bread and Roses from Stones*, wrote that our first consideration should be the quality of our crops and their nutritive value: "Certainly no one in his senses would be satisfied with a large harvest poor in food value, or deficient in essential minerals, because neither man nor beast can thrive on such food." Have we lost our senses? Why eat things that are unfit to serve as food? We've been trying to do that for a good many years. Should we wonder why we are deficient in so many nutrients?

On the other hand, organic fertilizers (compost, manure, rock dust, seaweed, fish meal, and the like) feed the soil which can then feed the plants. The plants are healthier, contain more nutrients, and can better resist disease. Pests are less of a problem and can be handled in nontoxic ways. Microorganisms thrive since the foods they need—the sugars, proteins, amino acids, minerals, and growth factors—are produced and made available as end-products by the decomposition of organic compounds (compost). William A Albrecht, a brilliant scientist, said that the plant "always eats at the second sitting, since the plant only gets what the microbe gives it." The true productivity of soil depends on the number, activity, and balance of soil microorganisms.

The fascinating story of soils, plants, and animals, as it relates to foods, is long and amazing. We have messed up the intricate ecology so much that our health, and the health of all the planet's inhabitants, is threatened.

Take herbicides, for example. They kill weeds by reducing the production of carotenes (like beta-carotene), vitamin E, and certain amino acids (building blocks of protein). The crops may not die, but they have poorer protein quality and fewer nutrients than they should.

When data from more than 100,000 government pesticide tests between 1992 and 2001 were analyzed, 192 different residues were detected on foods. Some foods contained many, others fewer. The word "pesticide" is similar to "homicide" or "suicide" because it indicates death or killing. Although pesticides are supposed to kill only "pests" of the plants (insects, animals, fungi, or weeds), plenty of animal tests and human statistics show that they are poisonous to everything, including us. Cancer, asthma and other respiratory diseases, damage to the nervous system (including Parkinson's disease), damage to the reproductive system, hormonal imbalances, birth defects, and many other ills are attributed to such toxic chemicals.

Animals, birds, and fish raised for food are commonly subject to unnatural conditions and fed unnatural pesticide-laden foods. They are unhealthy, given drugs, and sacrificed before they die from being sick. Their flesh does not contain the nutrients found in healthy, naturally-raised critters. Actually, the accumulation of pesticide-, hormone-, and drug-residues makes them more toxic than plant foods farmed with chemicals.

Add to this the chemicals used in processing many nonfoods (solvents, fumigants, humectants, bleaches, emulsifiers, texturizers, anti-caking and free-flowing agents, artificial flavors and colors, chemical preservatives, petroleum by-products, and many more) as well as the plastics and aluminum used in packaging from which chemicals migrate into food.

We may be told that "a little bit won't hurt you," and that "everything's fine in moderation." But, the accumulation of many small hits from toxic chemicals like pesticides or preservatives creates or contributes to big problems, including the chronic degenerative diseases that are now rampant. It's not the small single dose, but the amount of cumulative exposure that is harmful.

This includes consumption of things we may eat that are artificial, nonfood in the true sense of the word. Take aspartame, for example, better known as NutraSweet or Equal. We're told that it does not damage brain function even though complaints relating to the nervous system are common. Yet, if you look inside brain/nerve cells, you would find that aspartame causes changes that affect neurotransmitters (chemical messengers). Olestra is fake fat. Not only will it skew digestive processes and give you runny diarrhea, but it interferes with absorption of fat-soluble vitamins like A, D, E, K, and essential fatty acids.

If you have not yet become anxious and tense, there's more. Some food items, such as spices, seasonings, meats, poultry, fruits, wheat, potatoes, and dry vegetable substances, may be irradiated. This means short-term exposure of food to electromagnetic radiation. Does this harm the food? For example, just as radiation therapy given to cancer patients depletes vitamin B_{12} and vitamin D from their bodies, food irradiation depletes B vitamins and fat-soluble vitamins like A and E. Like human radiation, food irradiation has been shown to alter cell structures and intracellular activity. "Free radicals" are produced, causing increased rancidity (oxidation) of unsaturated fats in cell membranes. Damage to cellular structures may occur. Changes in membrane permeability to electrolytes are evident. There are many "problematic effects" that occur in living tissues. Raw fruits and vegetables and other raw or uncooked real foods are living tissues. Even if they are later cooked, the "problematic effects" have already taken place.

Then there is the advent of genetically engineered (GE) crops. More than 30 GE crops have been approved for sale in the US. From 60% to 80% of foods (mostly processed foods) in grocery stores contain at least some GE ingredients. GE soy and corn are often used to feed livestock. Genetic modification means that genes from one organism are transferred to another in ways that don't occur in Nature. It's complicated, unpredictable, and scary. Too much is unknown about mix-n'-match gene play, but we're learning the hard way. Scientists are manipulating Nature without knowing what they are doing or what the outcome may be.

It's claimed that GE crops reduce the need for pesticides (including herbicides and fungicides). But many GE crops are designed to be more resistant to pesticides so more can be used. More pesticides have been used since GE crops were introduced. It's claimed that GE crops will be good for the environment, but toxins from them kill insects other than "pests," such as butterflies, moths, beetles, lacewings, and others. The toxins seep into the soil and can stay active for seven or eight months. GE pollen gets washed into streams and underground water. Some of the "weeds" that are killed include herbs, wildflowers, important sources of fodder, plants that attract beneficial insects or microorganisms, sources of soil nutrients, or toxin removers, among others.

Some maintain that GE concoctions such as rBST—recombinant bovine somatotropin, a growth hormone—will translate to healthier milk and meat animals. But rBST unnaturally boosts milk output in cows, producing severe mastitis and other problems for the animals and hormone residues in their milk. A GE-derived rennet substitute is used in more than 50% of US cheeses. GE crops are fed to livestock, creating even more problems. Hogs have birthing problems; cows stop eating or even die.

Anothe dubious assessment is that GE plants will stay put, but the pollen spreads across the country and cross-pollination occurs over large distances. Weeds may acquire traits from pesticide-resistant plants, creating super weeds and the need for stronger pesticides. Corn, canola, and soybeans have been hopelessly contaminated. Altered genes may permanently change genetic codes of any number of other organisms. It's claimed that GE crops will feed the hungry, but there has been no significant difference in crop yields. The safety of GM crops can't be ensured. They are definitely not cheaper or of higher quality, and they won't solve world hunger.

Since GE foods entered the marketplace in 1996, more and more foods in the supermarket contain genetically-modified (GM) ingredients. They have not been tested for human safety, and animal testing "was woefully short and inadequate." Many scientists warn that they have the potential to cause health problems such as hormonal disruptions, allergies, toxicity, poisoning, birth defects, and cancer. GE foods contribute to immune dysfunction and they produce alien proteins. They may be toxic to the liver and kidneys, increase blood sugar levels, and cause mineral loss. Some harmful effects may not be obvious for years because of the gradual development of disease.

Others claim that GM foods can have more nutrients and better taste, but this is not occurring either. Nutrient parts, rather than the whole package, are being genetically plugged in, and, even though the products are called "functional foods," they're not helping health. Actually, the more that foods are genetically engineered, the lower their *real* nutritional value. Concentrations of some nutrients are lower, and it's not clear whether humans can actually absorb the GE nutrients. No thanks. I'll trust Nature.

Tests show that our bodies house numerous toxic chemicals, especially those obtained from "foods" we eat. In fact, the prevalence of toxins in US adults is often so high that reference ranges have been set for "allowable" levels, which include several dozen pesticide residues. For instance, toxins from foods have been shown to affect each and every process in the body that gets disrupted during the development of cancer.

Modern agribusiness procedures have caused a huge loss of nutrients from our foods and added a huge amount of toxins to the food, soil, water, and air. Our bodies try to detoxify, to get rid of as much of the junk as possible, but they can't handle the deluge. Toxic chemicals play a big role in malnutrition, in not getting the nutrients our bodies need to function well. Some folks may indeed eat what we might consider a decent diet that should supply plenty of nutrients, yet they are not protected from degeneration or disease because of their toxic load. Plus, detoxification itself requires a vast array of food-derived nutrients.

Did you know that representatives from many pharmaceutical (drug) companies sit on the boards of directors of numerous food companies, or that just about every drug company owns patents related to food production? We modern-day consumers are supposed to have more awareness of diet and nutrition than ever before, yet we seem to have been increasingly removed from the food supply processes. We assume that there can't be much wrong with food items on grocery shelves, but this is not true. It's up to us to either find out what we are eating or at least avoid any item that we are not sure about. I have often told clients to read labels for ingredients and, for example, if you can't pronounce it, don't eat it.

It is well worth noting that all of these things that are done to foods either decrease the nutrients or increase our need for more nutrients.

The use of toxic chemicals, the over-processing and adulterating and mangling of popular foods, and the disregard for nutritional value are among the factors that reflect the truth that, in the name of health, the issue of wholeness must be addressed. The whole spectrum of agricultural practices, manufacturing practices, lifestyle, and eating habits must be taken into account when we consider food. The philosophical root for all malnutrition and all toxicity is disregard for wholeness. It's this neglect that brings with it depletion, disruption, dysfunction, and disease.

According to Joel Kimmons, a nutritional expert for the Centers for Disease Control (CDC), "The US has the highest level of malnutrition in the world."

References:
Challam, Jack, "Genetically Modified Corn Results in Significant Biochemical Changes," *Alternative & Complementary Therapies*, June 2007: 13(3):167, citing GE Seralini, D Cellier, et al, "New Analysis of a Rat Feeding Study with a Genetically Modified Maize Reveals Signs of Hepatorenal Toxicity," *Archives of Environmental Contamination and Toxicology*, 2007: 52:596-602.
DeCava, Judith A. "Genetic Engineering and Food," *Nutrition News and Views*, Sept./Oct. 2004: 8(5):1-6, and "The Worth of Organic Foods," *Nutrition News and Views*, May/June 2005: 9(3):3.
"Fruits, Vegetables Less Nutritious Than 50 Years Ago," *Acres USA,* Aug. 2006: 36(8):9.

"Harvesting Health from the Garden," *Acres USA*, Nov. 2006: 36(11):69.

Johnson, Jean, "Kicking the White Stuff," *Environmental Magazine*, July/Aug. 2007: 18(4):42-43.

Levin, Buck, *Environmental Nutrition*, Vashon Island, WA: HingePin Integrative Learning Materials, 1999.

"Pesticide Tests Reveal the Most Contaminated Produce," *True Health,* Jan./Feb. 2004: 6.

Quesnell, William R., "Eating the 'Right Foods' Does Not Prevent Disease," *Health and Healing Wisdom*, Summer 2007: 31(2):13.

Worthington, Virginia, "Nutritional Quality of Organic Versus Conventional Fruits, Vegetables, and Grains," *Journal of Alternative and Complementary Medicine*, 2001: 7(2):161-173.

FOOD FOR THOUGHT

What benefit do we get from gigantic industrial farms? Cheap, readily available food. What are the consequences? That's a long, sad, complicated story. I could write a whole book about that. There are environmental and human health issues that affect you and me.

"Remember," says biochemist Harold N. Simpson, "artificial fertilizers are the junk foods of the plants."

Reference: Simpson, Harold N. *Unhealthy Food=Unhealthy People*, Chicago: Peter Jon Simpson, 1994:59.

A team of scientists has determined that the widespread use of synthetic nitrogen fertilizers and pesticides over the past 40 years has resulted in reducing plant yield by about one-third. We're getting less food and more toxins from the farms. Is there something wrong with this picture?

Reference: *Acres USA*, "Pesticides Reduce Crop Yields," *Acres USA,* Sept. 2007: 37(9):10.

"Human life is much more important than shelf life."

Reference: Lynne D Richardson, a member of the New York City Board of Health, on the city's current plan to limit restaurants' use of trans fats.

"A hundred years ago you wouldn't need a detective—or a journalist—to tell you what you were eating. But now it takes a lot of investigative journalism to find out what's in that Twinkie."

Reference: Black, Jane, "Food Detective," *Food & Wine*, Aug. 2006: 108.

"Don't eat anything your great-grandmother wouldn't recognize as food. Think about that when you pick up that tube of Go-Gurt. Would she know how to administer that?"

Reference: Michael Pollan, author of *The Omnivore's Dilemma*, on choosing whole-some, nutritious foods, cited in *Eating Well*, Sept./Oct. 2007: 6(5):14.

An analysis of 111 studies of soft drinks, juice, and milk "suggests" that research funding plays a definite role in nutrition studies. Studies funded by the beverage industry, for example, were 4 to 8 times more likely to be favorable to the interests of the funders than other research. In other words, we must ask where the money to fund the study comes from.

Reference: "Origin of Funding Seems to Influence Which Studies Are Done," *Tufts University Health & Nutrition Letter*, Mar. 2007: 25(1):3.

When sugars and amino acids in carbohydrate foods (like grains and potatoes) are subjected to high temperatures in cooking, a chemical called acrylamide is formed. Acrylamide is potentially carcinogenic. Depleted soil nutrition contributes to the problem. One study found that low sulfur content in soils leads to low sulfur in wheat and high acrylamide levels when it is cooked at high temperatures. Unexpectedly high levels of acrylamide were found in a wide range of heat-processed foods such as crackers, biscuits, and crisp breads. So, not only do you get cheated of nutrients when soils are depleted by modern farming methods, but you get more toxins.

Reference: "Acrylamide in Low-sulfur Wheat," *Acres USA,* Jan. 2007, 37(1):10.

Have you seen some milk products that don't have to be kept refrigerated? That's because of ultra-high temperature (UHT) processing. The milk is heated to at least 280° F for a few seconds. Traditional pasteurization heats milk to 161°F for 15 seconds or so—to kill bacteria, though it also destroys enzymes and nutrients. The UHT process goes further and destroys any spores that cause spoilage which may be left in the milk. (You still have to refrigerate the milk after you open the container.) The flavor is changed enough to make me believe that other not-so-healthy alterations have taken place as well, including the mangling of other nutrients.

Reference: "No Fridge for UHT Milk?," *Environmental Nutrition,* Sept. 2007, 30(9):7.

Many wild varieties of wheat were found to have higher concentrations of protein, iron, and zinc than domesticated wheat. As humans domesticated wheat, the health benefits decreased. Domestication included messing with genetic tendencies. It seems to me that, every time humans mess with Nature, they mess themselves.

Reference: "Wheat Gone Wild," *Science News,* 9 Dec. 2006: 170(24):382.

Don't eat the citrus peels of any citrus fruits—including the zests of orange and lime that are often grated—unless they are organically grown. Citrus crops in the US are routinely sprayed with several pesticides, a number of which are carcinogenic, which tend to remain in the skin.

Reference: Bader, Myles H., *2001 Food Secrets Revealed*, Las Vegas NV: Northstar Publishing, 1997: 65.

WHAT HAPPENED TO OUR FOOD?

About 50% of all the antibiotics manufactured in this country are used on animals—chickens, pigs, and cattle. The animals are frequently sick because of being cooped up, questionable sanitary conditions, unnatural feeds, and stress. Not only are the animals becoming antibiotic resistant, but many scientists believe that humans are becoming antibiotic resistant because of eating the meats of the antibiotic-treated animals. I have a low tolerance for mistreatment of animals—it makes me livid. And I have a low tolerance for mistreatment of human beings who don't even realize that they are being mistreated.

Reference: Dr Myles H Bader, Myles H., *2001 Food Secrets Revealed*, Las Vegas NV: Northstar Publishing, 1997: 106-107.

Genetic engineering is like playing genetic roulette with inherited traits. Take, for example, the cauliflower mosaic virus which is used to infect the embryo or seed of plants. This virus carries a little genetic combination which is wanted in a plant. As the virus invades and spreads throughout the developing plant, it "infects" the plant with this new genetic trait. Monsanto has done this with its herbicide-resistant soybeans and other plants. The herbicide doesn't kill these plants—it's retained within the plants. When animals or humans eat the food from such plants, the herbicide is released and adversely affects intestinal bacteria. It can cause irritable, inflammatory bowel problems among other things.

Crops that have been genetically engineered are causing systemic (throughout the body) damage, especially to our immune systems. All your body knows is that it is receiving foreign proteins—proteins that were never around before and don't belong in our bodies. Is it any wonder that there are more illnesses due to immune compromises or collapse? What about the increased number of people with allergies, chemical and food sensitivities, so-called "autoimmune" diseases, even cancer?

Reference: Fox, Michael W., "Eco-ethics for a Healthy Planet," *Acres USA*, Aug. 2007: 37(8):56-61.

Chapter Three

WHAT ABOUT HISTORY?

That's a long story. There's not enough room in this little book to go all the way through the history of nutrition, so I'll whisk through a few facts to make a point.

We're told that we have better health and that we are living longer than at any other time in history. It's nice to believe that, but it's not exactly true. Yes, humans have come a long way. There is a more steady supply of food—for some of us, but definitely not all peoples on earth—than during other periods of history. The statistics seem to indicate that we are living longer. But, you know about lies and statistics.

Truth is, the US ranks only 16th in life span. Yet this country is one of the most technologically advanced nations, with more food available to more people, and, supposedly, one of the best health care systems. US citizens are not really living much longer than they used to. You've seen the numbers, that in 1900 the average life expectancy was 45 years. Now it's about 75 years. The 30-year increase is almost entirely due to a reduction in infant mortality. When you remove infant deaths from the equation, life expectancy has only increased 3.7 years over the last 100 years. Historians also point to improvements in sanitation for reducing many "infectious" diseases and other illnesses.

The reality is that younger people are failing and dying at earlier ages than their grandparents. A considerable number of folks who live past the age of 100 are in better condition than many of their grandchildren. The 20th century saw the burgeoning of what are called degenerative diseases: long-term, enduring, gradually deteriorating, devastating conditions. These include heart disease, arthritis, diabetes, asthma and other respiratory problems, multiple sclerosis, cancers of all types, and many others. More than 100 years ago, folks had no inkling of our "modern" conditions like multiple chemical sensitivity or food allergies and intolerances. This and the previous generation are the first to be exposed to a plethora of poisons and toxins continuously throughout their lives. That's a major reason for unhealthiness. Another aspect of declining health is that people engage in much less physical activity than they used to. The loss of community and spiritual values has also been cited as still another explanation. But a really big problem is one of nutrition; actually the lack of it. Too many people in this and other developed countries are starving and don't know it. Many of them are actually overweight or obese, but they haven't been and aren't getting the nutrients they need to be healthy.

Yes, refined sugar was made back in the Middle ("Dark") Ages, but was available only to the very rich. Health was not a strong point during that period of history. People of means looked upon vegetables and fruit as peasant food and avidly avoided them. Sanitation was non-existent. I am digressing. The point is that refining (stripping off the nutrient-dense parts of foods), over-processing, and chemical adulteration of foods really became widespread during the 1900s and is still expanding and evolving. Scientists can create just about anything in their labs that looks good enough to eat and may even taste good, but has lost semblance to being real food. It's time to get back to basics, and I'm not the first or only one who thinks so.

Numerous health activists and nutrition pioneers over the last 100 years or so have courageously spoken out about the dangers of what had and is being done to our food. I can't possibly mention them all. There was Weston A Price, DDS, a dentist who traveled around the world during the 1930s to compare "primitive" (traditional) and "modern" (refined, processed) diets. He was, of course, especially interested in the condition of the people's teeth, but he found that, in addition to good strong teeth, the native peoples who ate local foods raised with love and respect for Nature—foods their people ate traditionally, fresh and whole—also enjoyed good health in every other aspect. Those who had "defected" to a modern diet of stripped, over-processed, often stale or rancid fabrications, had decayed, missing, unhealthy teeth along with all sorts of illnesses and diseases, including heart disease and cancer.

Dr Francis M. Pottenger, Jr., who, between the years 1932 and 1942, conducted an experiment with some 900 cats, comparing a diet of raw meat and raw milk with that of cooked meat and cooked (pasteurized) milk. The cats on the cooked foods developed arthritis and other problems of bones, muscles, teeth or other structures, under or over-activity of glands like the thyroid or ovaries or testes, inflammation of the nervous system with paralysis and meningitis, abnormal respiratory tissues with bronchitis and lung conditions, heart disease, problems during pregnancy, had stillbirths or delivery problems during birth, more irritability and aggression or more passivity and docility, among other maladies. The cats fed raw meat and milk thrived, showed every sign of health from their bone structure to their fur, were more resistant to inflammation, fleas and other parasites, were friendly and playful. Even though we humans are not cats, the study did prove that the foods and nutrients needed by each species are essential to good health.

Dr. William Albrecht, of the University of Missouri, showed that the nutritional quality of foods for humans and animals raised on deficient soils, with chemical fertilizers, and later, treated with various pesticides and herbicides, was increasingly declining. He and others stressed that we have been losing track of the fundamentals of good nutrition.

Dr. Robert McCarrison studied and wrote about the connection between nutritional deficiencies and various diseases as well as the symptoms of specific deficiencies. His book, *Studies in Deficiency Disease*, was published in 1921.

What was so outstanding about all these people and what they advocated? They were courageous people who told the truth in the face of contrary medical and agricultural beliefs of the time. During the earlier years of the 20th century, it was believed that basically only germs (like bacteria and later, viruses) caused disease. It was thought that nutrition had nothing to do with disease except the few obvious problems that developed when severe deficiency existed; problems like scurvy, beriberi, pellagra, and rickets. It was believed that artificial stimulation of plant and animal growth by chemical fertilizers and ridding plants of insects or weeds by miracle chemicals was better than the old farming methods. Who thought about what it did to the nutritional and health value of the foods when chemicals could cure just about everything? Only some brave, independent thinkers who were concerned about the health of others.

No one vied in the face of these skewed scientific claims more than Dr. Royal Lee. He understood and knew that the North American food supply was suffering because of refining, processing, chemical farming, chemical additives and the like. In 1929 he formulated his first nutritional supplement, Catalyn, to make up for some of the nutrients that were low or missing from common foods. It was basically a concentrate of real foods. The effects of Catalyn were so impressive, so helpful to people with a number of diseases or illnesses—some considered incurable at that time—that in 1933 Dr. Lee wrote about its effectiveness to show how important nutrition was to healing and health. He was condemned by the FDA (Food and Drug Administration) and other scientific bodies. By 1939 more than 90% of the diseases that he had listed as being helped by Catalyn were then known to be caused or aggravated by nutritional deficiencies. Dr. Lee was condemned for saying that foods and their nutrients were therapeutic or healing. My grandmother and herbalist great-grandmother knew this long before scientists realized it. Your grandparents and other ancestors did too. They knew that wholesome, real foods were needed for health, that whole herbs and foods would help the body to heal.

Dr. Lee went on to promote clean, wholesome, naturally-raised foods, to make more food supplements, and to expose the toxic, nutrient-draining, devitalizing, mangling interference of commercial enterprises. He stressed that "you can't make something out of nothing." We need nutrient-dense foods. He fumed over the lies that people were told and he prolifically wrote articles and printed the research and evidence. For telling the truth, he was persecuted and prosecuted. Dr. Lee said that he spent 98% of his time battling with someone to make him/her believe the facts on which his work was based and only 2% of his time developing new and useful products to help people. The original name of his supplement business, Therapeutic Food Company, did not stand the scrutiny of the FDA because foods were not considered to be therapeutic. According to the FDA and others, humans would never need supplements if they ate a well-balanced diet, and that there was no such thing as junk food. In 1939, FDA authorities insisted that there is no human disease or illness possible from any vitamin or mineral deficiency in the diet. (US Court of Appeals, 7th Circuit 6867, 1939) In 1949 (US District Court, DC Civil Action No.5208-48) an FDA expert under oath stated that no proof was available to show that a well-fed person was less likely to incur disease than one less well fed. The consensus of medical opinion was more important than proving that nutrient-dense whole foods were essential to health.

Dr. Lee lamented the declining value of industrialized foods and supplements. He spoke of the floods of counterfeit foods in the markets that took a terrible toll in human health and happiness. "Counterfeit foods are like counterfeit money," he said. "They drive good foods (or good money) out of circulation." These days we are even more deluged with nonfoods and have to seek out honest-to-goodness real food.

V. Earl Irons, founder of a nutritional supplement firm that made real food concentrates, stated in lectures that most people in this country were suffering from malnutrition or were in danger of suffering because of the depletion of soils and the refining and processing of foods. He had volumes of scientific proof. But, for saying this, he was fined $6,000.00 and sentenced to a year in jail in 1957. The research from government and university sources did not conform to the "consensus of medical opinion." He went to prison for telling the truth. While he was in prison, there were three major food strikes by prisoners, making it necessary to move him from prison to prison. V. Earl Irons was quick to point out that the poor quality of food contributed to the dysfunction and behavior of people, thus creating more and more prisoners.

Dr. Lee, V. Earl Irons, and all the others persisted despite opposition. The nutritional company Dr. Lee established still thrives today (Standard Process, Inc.) and, although he died in 1967, his teachings continue to amaze and instruct doctors, nutritionists, and anyone interested in nutrition and disease. His work and writings inspired many to continue and add to his well-laid foundation.

Have things changed today? There has been progress, that's for sure. Ever so slowly, it is being established and accepted that nutrition and wholesome foods are essential for good health. It is accepted that nutrients and foods can prevent and help just about every disease condition there is. Still, there is a long way to go. There's a whole lot of foot-dragging. I can remember during the 1980s being told by some clients that their doctors insisted that nutrition has nothing to do with disease. Even now, diseases are often considered drug deficiencies. And, if nutrients have anything to do with health problems, then the rush is on to develop a means to convert them into drugs or drug-like substances.

Did you know that many registered dieticians still stand by the idea that anything you can put in your mouth without immediately collapsing is fine to eat—that there is no such thing as junk food? I heard one dietician say that she keeps Twinkies in her office to snack on, that she considers all "foods" in the same way. Just count calories and cut the amount of fat you eat. Makes me nauseous.

Anyone who is a nutritionist or other health practitioner using nutrition or herbs still cannot claim to cure or relieve disease or illness. Only medical doctors can do that with drugs or surgery or radiation. When any of my clients enthusiastically speak of how foods and food supplements "cured" or "healed" them or a loved one, I caution them that they cannot say that: it was simply a happy accident or pleasant side effect.

We must credit many of the pioneers listed above, along with many others, such as Dr. Harvey Wiley who served as chief chemist at the Department of Agriculture during the early 1900s until he was forced to resign in 1912 because he told the truth about the devitalization and adulteration of foods. Other pioneers include Rachel Carson, who began the expose on toxic chemicals, Dr. Henry G. Bieler, who successfully treated patients with real foods, and Beatrice Trum Hunter, who has written for decades about the problems with industrialized foods and the benefits of real foods. All these people with vision can be cited and credited with beginning and perpetuating the movement to understand what true nutrition is all about.

To all of them, mentioned or not, I say, "Thank you."

References:

Bieler, Henry G., *Food is Your Best Medicine*, New York: Ballantine Books, 1965.

Carson, Rachel, *Silent Spring*, Boston: Houghton Mifflin Company, 1962.

DeCava, Judith A., "Longevity," *Nutrition News and Views*, Sept./Oct. 2001: 5(5):1-10.

Hunter, Beatrice Trum, *Additives Book*, New Canaan, CT: Keats Publishing, Inc., 1972: along with numerous other books and articles she has written.

Lectures of Dr. Royal Lee, 2 volumes, reproduced and published by Selene River Press, Fort Collins, CO: 1998 & 1999.

Lee, Royal, *Vitamin News*—a compilation of newsletters from 1933 to 1956: reproduced and published by the International Foundation for Nutrition & Health, San Diego, CA.

Maguelonne Toussaint-Samat, Maguelonne, *History of Food*, translated by Anthea Bell, New York: Barnes & Noble, Inc, 1992.

McCarrison, Robert, *Studies in Deficiency Disease*, London: Henry Frowde and Hodder & Stoughton, 1921: reproduced by the Lee Foundation for Nutritional Research in 1945.

Murray, Richard P., *Reflections of a Genius,* 1990: unpublished compilation of quotations, correspondence, and writings of Dr. Royal Lee and those who knew him.

Natenberg, Maurice, *The Legacy of Doctor Wiley*, Chicago: Regent House, 1957.

Pottenger, Francis M. Jr., *Pottenger's Cats: A Study in Nutrition*, edited by Elaine Pottenger, La Mesa, CA: Price-Pottenger Nutrition Foundation, Inc., 1995 edition.

Price, Weston A., *Nutrition and Physical Degeneration*, New Canaan, CT: Keats Publishing, Inc., 1989: originally published in 1945.

Trager, James, *The Food Chronology*, New York: Henry Holt and Company, 1995.

FOOD FOR THOUGHT

The diets of our early human ancestors have been difficult to completely determine. But recent evidence shows that they probably had quite a diverse diet—varying with the seasons—and which, in some areas, included animals feeding on grasses. Grass-fed animals were and are extremely nutritious.

> Reference: Sponheimer, Matt, Benjamin H. Passey, et al, "Isotopic Evidence for Dietary Variability in the Early Hominim *Paranthropus Robustus*, *Science*, 10 Nov. 2006: 314(5801):980-981.

The primitive Eskimos, despite living in a frigid climate, never suffered from arthritis and other chronic or degenerative diseases. They ate large amounts of raw food. The meat they ate was only partially-cooked and was raw in the center. Thus, the Eskimo consumed a lot of enzymes which are part of nutrient complexes and which give nutrients a life energy. In fact, the word "Eskimo" comes from an expression meaning, "He who eats it raw."

> Reference: Howell, Edward, *Food Enzymes for Health & Longevity*, Twin Lakes WI: Lotus Press, 1994: 20.

Back in the late 1950s, there was a legal case that, today, would seem ludicrous. One of the pioneers of real nutrition, Dr. Royal Lee, was forbidden by the Food and Drug Administration (FDA) to continue using the name Therapeutic Food Company for his business. Why? Because food was not considered to be therapeutic, not healing.

During a lecture on January 12, 1951, Dr Royal Lee lamented that: "One of the biggest tragedies of human civilization is the precedence of chemical therapy over nutrition. It's a substitution of artificial therapy over natural, of poisons over food, in which we are feeding people poisons in trying to correct the reactions of starvation." I wish I could say that things have changed, but there is certainly a glimmer of hope in that many people are becoming wiser. We are gradually working our way back to Nature.

> Reference: Lee, Royal, *Lectures of Dr. Royal Lee*, Fort Collins CO: Selene River Press, 1998: VII.

Dr. Weston A. Price and other writers on malnutrition who made exhaustive studies of peoples in various nations stress the point that in areas or in groups where "civilized" nonfoods were not used, there was very little or almost no heart disease, cancer, arthritis, tuberculosis, pneumonia, and tooth decay. In some cases, the number of dental cavities ranged from 0 to less than 1%. Dr. Price even noted that the "primitive" people living on their traditional diets did not suffer from appendicitis, gallbladder trouble, cystitis, or duodenal ulcers. They were usually known for their physical strength and endurance as well as their good minds. Traditionally, they knew to obtain foods that sometimes were scarce, but were rich in certain elements required for good health. Dr. Price stressed the need to "return to harmony with Nature's laws, since life in its fullness is Nature obeyed."

Reference: Price, Weston A., *Nutrition and Physical Degeneration*, New Canaan CT (Keats Publishing Inc), 1989.

Dr. Royal Lee often explained that "you do not need to be an expert in nutrition to get good food. You just have to be hard-boiled enough to say 'no' when you are offered a food that is unfit to eat." Wish I'd said that.

Lee, Royal, address to "United Farmers of America," 7 Dec. 1949, *Lectures of Dr. Royal Lee*, Fort Collins CO: Selene River Press, 1998: 85.

Dr. Bieler had a broth recipe that became somewhat famous to support energy, weight loss, and detoxification. Here's the basic recipe, adapted from his book, *Food is Your Best Medicine*:

- 3 stalks of celery
- 3 whole zucchini
- 2 cups of string beans
- 1 cup of parsley

Put 1 cup of good, clean water in a stock pot. Then put in the string beans and steam for about 5 minutes. Add the celery and zucchini; steam for another 5 to 7 minutes (or until tender but still crisp). Don't overcook. When the vegetables are tender, drain the water from the pot (that the veggies cooked in) into a blender. Then follow with the cooked vegetables. Blend until liquefied. Add a teaspoon or so of raw unsalted butter and the parsley. Blend again until the parsley is liquefied. Enjoy.

- Optional: add 1 clove of garlic, minced, with the string beans and cook with the vegetables.

Chapter Four

WHAT DO WE DO NOW?

Food defines a culture. I have to ask myself, what do the things people eat in the US say about our culture? Ding Dongs? Super-sized? Deep-fried Mars Bars? Hot Pockets? Frosted Flakes? Seriously, I'd say there is bad news and good news. There is tremendous pressure to submit to the industrialized, profit-seeking, health-compromising food market. Then there is a growing trend for celebrating food as a labor of love, a source of being in touch with Nature and our own bodies, a true source of nourishment and vitality. People increasingly want, and need, wholesome, healthful, nutrient-dense real foods. Don't you?

Think about what John Neustadt, ND stated: "The prevalence of chronic, degenerative diseases attributable wholly or in part to dietary patterns is the most serious threat to public health in the United States." He said that what we eat has a tremendous influence on our health or lack of health. Some of the degenerative diseases that are greatly influenced by foods and nutrition (nonfoods and nutritional deficits) include cardiovascular disease (CVD), cancer, type 2 diabetes, arthritis, and overweight/obesity.

One third of North American adults (that's more than 71 million people) have some form of CVD, the number-one cause of death. CVD accounted for 37.3% of all US deaths in 2003. It was "an underlying or contributing cause" for about 58% of deaths in 2002, according to the American Heart Association. The number-two cause of mortality is cancer, causing 25% of US deaths. Scientific research has indicated that at least one-third of all cancer deaths are attributable to poor nutrition, physical inactivity, and overweight or obesity. These same risk factors may account for up to 80% of colon, breast, and prostate cancers. About 65% of American adults are now classified as overweight or obese, with the numbers still growing. Almost a third of American children are at risk for or already are overweight or obese. Obesity (being grossly overweight) contributes to more than 280,000 deaths every year in the US.

So what do we do?

We become educated about food, at least a little, so we know what we are consuming. The answer, I believe, to the quest for the wholly grail—whole, real, nutrient-dense food—is organic farming. Organic food means reclaiming influence on our health, our children's health, and the earth's health. For a while, the emphasis for organic farming was on avoiding the poisons and toxins. Now, thank goodness, there is also more importance being placed on building the soil and working with Nature, rather than trying to control or manipulate it, so that the food produced contains more nutrients and other good stuff.

We should be eating high-quality, nutrient-dense foods, but modern industrial agribusinesses aren't giving it to us. The USDA (US Department of Agriculture) has the statistics that show nutrient density has been dropping, a lot. Declines in nutrients like protein, calcium, phosphorus, iron, vitamin B_2, vitamin C, and many others range anywhere from 6% to 38%. Use of synthetic fertilizers, use of pesticides (including herbicides and fungicides), use of hybrid seeds, and other "modern" farming methods are responsible for much of this decrease. Organic farming is showing that it is not only possible to reverse that trend, but that it is already happening on many organic farms.

Organic farming is much better for the environment because it contributes to preserving wildlife habitats, safeguarding and replenishing topsoil, generally improving the quality of the soil, and supporting rather than disrupting the ecology, among other attributes. Organic composts, made from aged plant and animal wastes, can actually break down pesticides and other toxic chemicals in the environment so that organic agriculture may actually help clean things up. Also, the effects of organic farming have a direct impact on human health by supplying cleaner water, cleaner air, the absence of pesticide and drug and hormone residues, lower levels of toxic heavy metals, better protein, no irradiation, no genetic engineering, and increasingly, more nutrients. These results apply to plant foods and animal foods.

So far, more than 40 studies show that organically-raised foods contain larger amounts of nutrients. Other studies show that they have more balanced amounts of nutrients and, in some cases, nutrients that were hardly known to exist in "conventionally-raised" foods.

One study showed that organic crops had, on average, up to 30% more vitamin C, iron, magnesium, and phosphorus. Another found that organically grown food was, on average, 63% higher in calcium, 73% higher in iron, 118% higher in magnesium, 178% higher in molybdenum (don't try to pronounce this trace mineral without help), 91% higher in phosphorus, 125% higher in potassium, and 60% higher in zinc. The organic food was, on average 29% lower in toxic mercury than conventionally-raised food. Still another scientific study stated that organically grown corn, strawberries, and marionberries had much higher levels of antioxidants than conventionally-grown versions. A look at apples revealed that the organic fruits contained more minerals like phenols, selenium, fibers, and vitamins C and E. Two independent comprehensive studies compared the differences between organic and conventional foods by analyzing about 40 previously published studies. They both found that there is overwhelming evidence that organic food is more nutritious than conventional food.

An Australian government agency found that organic foods have up to 10 times more mineral content than conventional produce. A 10-year comparison of tomatoes raised organically and conventionally showed that phytochemical flavonoids (quercetin and kaempferol) were 79% and 97% higher in the organic items. Kiwi fruits grown organically contain more concentrated levels of minerals and higher amounts of vitamin C and phenols than those grown conventionally. Organically-grown potatoes have higher levels of vitamin C than conventionally-grown spuds. Many studies also find that a variety of organically produced vegetables—particularly dark, leafy greens like chard, kale, and spinach—have higher levels of vitamin C. *No* studies showed that organic foods had lower nutrient levels than conventionally-raised versions. Several studies showed differences in nutrient levels in organic milk and cheese. For example, the organic types had higher levels of vitamin E, beta-carotene, and omega-3 fatty acids. More studies are needed to learn about differences in other nutrients in these foods.

Nevertheless, historical records from the USDA certainly show that common fruits and vegetables today contain lower amounts of nutrients than did their predecessors. All the minerals studied in wheat have declined, for example. Although reliance on chemicals and close plant spacing tend to produce fast-growing, high-yielding plants, these plants often have poorly-developed root systems that can't absorb the quantity of many nutrients that well-developed root systems will. Additionally, the use of synthetic fertilizers has resulted in lower nutrient content in the soils so that plants don't have enough to begin with.

Organic foods can give you some or a lot more nutrition. They're worth finding and buying because it's your health and your family's health we're talking about.

The last chapter mentioned how the huge amount of nitrogen chemicals in artificial fertilizers makes plants increase protein production and decrease carbohydrate production. The glitch is that the protein is poor quality. Organically-managed soils release nitrogen in smaller amounts over a longer period of time. The quantity of protein in organic grains and vegetables is lower, but the quality, in terms of human nutrition, is much, much better.

A review of scientific studies led nutritionist Shane Heaton to conclude, "Unless you eat organic, one item in three in your fridge or kitchen cupboard is likely to have chemical residues which often occur in potentially dangerous combinations." Modern-day farming means using pesticides. The FDA estimates that 20 pounds of pesticides are used per person each year. At least 50 of these pesticides are classified as carcinogenic (cancer causing). Conventional farming—the way foods are commonly raised in the US—entails the use of numerous pesticides which include herbicides, insecticides, fungicides, and other chemicals.

When you eat conventional vegetables and fruits, pesticides and chemicals tend to show up in your body. Eating the 12 most contaminated fruits and vegetables exposes a person to an average of 15 pesticides a day. (The 12 worst offenders or "dirty dozen" are peaches, apples, bell peppers, celery, nectarines, strawberries, cherries, pears, grapes, spinach, lettuce, and potatoes.) Peanuts are in the top 10 foods contaminated with persistent pollutants which build up in your fatty tissues. North Americans eat about 2.4 billion pounds of peanuts each year, about half in the form of peanut butter. Sadly, 85% of the 2004 soybean crop was genetically modified. From 2000 to 2005, more than 2,100 new foods containing soy appeared on the US market. Almost half of all corn planted in the US in 2004 was genetically modified. Corn is fed to meat animals and used to make corn sweeteners that appear in most processed foods. Cacao, used to make chocolate, is one of the world's most heavily pesticide-sprayed crops.

The European Union has banned the use of growth hormones for cattle, but these hormones are widely used in the US. The "food" that cattle eat (like manure and processed auto tires) would make you sick just to hear about. Organically-raised cattle eat organic feed, or even better, the grass they were meant to consume. In 2004, North Americans spent more than $70 billion on beef. The same use of drugs and disgusting feeds are used for pork and poultry. Hogs and poultry in the US are given about 20 million pounds of antibiotics every year (for contrast, about three million pounds are given to sick people). In a 2006 study, more than half the supermarket chicken samples tested positive for arsenic. Milk from cows given recombinant bovine growth hormone (rBGH), a synthetic drug given to cows to increase milk production, contains higher levels of a growth factor called IGF-1. Some scientists have linked excess levels of it in humans to breast and prostate cancers. The European Union has banned this drug. Use of rBGH in the US increases inflammations in cows, prompting the administering of even more antibiotics. Huge farms with 500 or more milk cows made up less than 4% of the number of dairy farms in 2004, but produced nearly half of the milk consumed in the US.

A DOZEN FOODS TO DEFINITELY BUY ORGANIC

1. **Meats:** Animals store high concentrations of chemicals (pesticides, drug, hormone, residues) in their fatty tissues, and some meats contain toxic additives. Worst: veal, bacon, deli meats, fast-food hamburgers, hotdogs, ground beef, liver, pork sausage.

2. **Dairy products:** They store harmful chemicals in their fats. Worst: butter, cream, cheese, half-and-half, ice cream, evaporated milk, processed cheese, whole milk.

3. **Fish:** Farmed fish frequently contain high levels of contaminants. Fish caught close to city harbors have high amounts of industrial pollutants and pesticides. Freshwater fish from polluted rivers and lakes are also contaminated. Large ocean fish, such as tuna, contain more mercury and other contaminants than small ocean fish.

4. **Berries:** Their very thin skins absorb harmful chemicals. **Raisins** are loaded with industrial chemical and pesticide residues.

5. **Mushrooms:** Powerful fungicides are used on them to extend shelf life. **Peanuts** often take the prize for the most pesticide-saturated plant food.

6. **Salad crops:** lettuce, spinach, bell peppers, and celery are highly sprayed.

7. **Root crops:** Carrots, beets, turnips, etc. absorb the chemicals sprayed on them.

8. **Waxed fruits and veggies:** The wax may contain fungicides and pesticides and it locks in other pesticides.

9. **Bananas:** They used to be pretty safe, but foreign plantations are often now using 20 times more pesticides than U.S. farms.

10. **Coffee and tea:** Brewing with hot water can concentrate residual pesticides. **Wine** has too many pesticides.

11. **French fries and frozen pizza:** Lots of pesticide residues. Pizza with meat has greater pesticide saturation in addition to nitrites.

12. **Miscellaneous:** Ready-to-eat cakes, many chocolate products, dill pickles, potato chips, soy oil and some soy products, partially-hydrogenated oils (trans fats).

(From *Living Green* by Greg Horn, Freedom Press Inc., and *Diet for a Poisoned Planet* by David Steinman, Harmony Books.)

Put succinctly, eat organic for what you *don't* get (chemical and drug residues, toxic metals, environmental harm, low nutrient value) and eat organic for what you *do* get (cleaner environment, far fewer or no toxins, often more nutrients, and definitely a more balanced nutrient value).

This brings to mind the disappearing honeybees. I'm sure you've heard that up to 60% of bees have disappeared. Why? There appear to be various reasons, though research still continues. One fairly new pesticide (clothianidin) could be a culprit, though other pesticides and herbicides may be involved. Electromagnetic radiation (as from cell phones), genetically-engineered crops, a virus, global warming, and other factors have also been suspected. Malnutrition seems to be a key player—bees are used on large agribusiness farms where the bees are used to pollinate one type of crop (mono-cropping), greatly limiting the nutrients that the bees get from that one (often chemically-sprayed and nutritionally-deficient) food. And places that used to have good plant forage for honeybees are shrinking because humans are destroying them with houses, freeways, and shopping malls. This subject could be a feature article by itself, perhaps in an issue of my newsletter, *Nutrition News and Views,* I will address it. But, what's happening to the bees may be a warning of what could befall humans. Some of the bees' symptoms include chronic fatigue, poor appetite, sluggish memory, signs of stress, and premature death. What about people? TV news programs frequently spotlight numerous human maladies of poor health including various degenerative diseases which have been linked to our accumulated toxic load as well as malnutrition. Like the bees, we seem to be getting *overwhelmed* by toxins and *undermined* by not getting enough of the real, whole food nutrients we need. Overfed but undernourished.

What do you do? Seek organic foods at supermarkets, health food stores, farmer's markets, and local farms. Join a co-op or a CSA (Community Supported Agriculture). Eat in-season if you can. Yes, it's worth the effort, time, and perhaps a little more money. If given the choice, go local for as many items as possible. They are often organically-raised, even if not certified (which is costly). You can always ask the farmer. You might find a dairy or creamery, source of eggs, winery, bakery, or other local businesses that go organic. Have a garden of your own. Plant fruit trees and berry bushes. About 75% of American consumers now buy at least some organic foods regularly. There are good reasons to buy organic for most, if not all, your food.

However, realize that the word "organic" is not magic. Organic junk food is still junk food minus a few toxins. Refined organic flour is still refined. Organic milled sugar is still refined sugar. Organic chips or cookies or French fries are still nonfoods. They won't give you the nutrients your body is asking for. Another caveat: there is tremendous pressure in the burgeoning organic industry to drive down prices and standards and import "cheap, dubious organic food" from places like China. Know the source and think.

Therefore, other than organic, the other thing we need to do is let our foods be as untampered-with as possible. Eat close to Nature, not industry. The more humans fool around with foods—the more they are stripped, mutilated, warped, defiled, configured, or simulated—the less value they have to your body. Eating such industrialized fabrications is definitely a case of diminishing returns. What's more important? Investing money into something that will financially support you in old age *or* investing wholesome, natural, real foods into good health that will better assure you will reach old age, and reach it with some vigor and vitality?

I hear some of you saying, "Wouldn't it be easier to just take supplements to make up for the nutrients I don't get in my food?" You probably already need to do that because of what you haven't been getting for most or all of your life. And we can't look at supplementation as another quick fix for all our problems. As Dr. Michael W. Fox wrote, "It is not supplementation, but *organic farming* that is the ultimate antidote and first medicine." Real whole foods are the foundation of good health and wellness. Supplements should do just what their name says—supplement an already good diet. It is unfortunate that we need to take supplements, but many of us do. If we have deficiencies, if we haven't received the best foods throughout our life, if we have some illness, disorder, or disease, we probably need the extra help from good supplements.

Ah, but what constitutes a good supplement? That's another chapter.

References:
"Another Score for Organics," *Body & Soul,* Nov./Dec. 2007: 24(8):26.

Burke, Cindy, *To Buy or Not to Buy Organic,* Da Capo Press, a member of the Perseus Book Group, 2007.

"Cancer Facts & Figures 2006," American Cancer Society. Secured pdf. http://www.cancer.org/downloads/STT/CAFF2006PW. Accessed 11 Apr. 2006.

Carmichael, Mary, "Organic Food and You," *Body & Soul,* Mar. 2007: 24(2):109-114.

Davis, Donald R., Melvin D. Epp, and Hugh D. Riordan, "Changes in USDA Food Composition Data for 43 Garden Crops, 1950 to 1999."

DeCava, Judith A., "The Worth of Organic Foods," *Nutrition News and Views,* May/June 2005: 9(3):1-6.

Fox, Michael W., "Organic Agriculture: First Medicine of Holistic Healing," *Acres USA,* July 2007: 37(7):72-75.

Frank, Jon C., "The Quest for Nutrient Density," *Acres USA,* June 2007,:37(6):76-77.

Glade, M.J., "Food, Nutrition, and the Prevention of Cancer: A Global Perspective," American Institute for Cancer Research/World Cancer Research fund, American Institute for Cancer Research, 1997." *Nutrition,* 1999: Vol.15, No.6, pp.523-526.

"Heart Disease and Stroke Statistics—2006 Update," American Heart Association. http://www.americanheart.org/downloadable/heart/1140534985281Statsupdate06book.pdf, Accessed 11 Apr. 2006.

"Higher Yield, Lower Nutrition," *Acres USA,* Nov. 2007: 37(11):10-11.

"How 'bout Them Apples," *Acres USA,* Feb. 2002: 32(2):7.

"Is Organic Food Really More Nutritious?," *Tufts University Health and Nutrition Letter,* Sept. 2007: 25(7):8.

Leu, Andre, "The Benefits of Organic Food," *Acres USA,* May 2004: 34(5):24-25.

Mitchel, Alyson E., Yun-Jeong Hong, et al, "Ten-year Comparison of the Influence of Organic and Conventional Crop Management Practices on the Content of Flavonoids in Tomatoes," *Journal of Agriculture and Food Chemistry,* epublished prior to print, 5 July 2007.

Mussen, Eric, "The Case of the Honeybee Killer," *Acres USA,* Nov. 2007: 37(11):56-63.

Neustadt, John, "Western Diet and Inflammation," *Integrative Medicine,* Aug./Sept. 2006: Vol.5, No.4, pp.14-18.

"Nutritional Value of Organics: Growing Evidence," *Health and Healing Widsom,* Summer 2002: 26(2):23, citing *Organic Farming, Food Quality and Human Health.*

"Organic Produce More Nutritious than Conventional, Says Australian Study," *Pesticides and You,* Spring 2000: 20(1):6-7.

"Organics 'R' Us," *Reader's Digest,* March 2007: p.228.

Worthington, Virginia, "Nutritional Quality of Organic Versus Conventional Fruits, Vegetables and Grains," *Journal of Alternative and Complementary Medicine*, 2001: 7(2):161-173, and in an interview, "Nutritional Quality: Organic vs. Conventional," *Clinical Pearls*, January 2002: 12(1):5-6.

FOOD FOR THOUGHT

Organic lettuce? Great. Organic meat? Terrific. But organic cotton candy? You can now get a certified organic version of the sweet sticky stuff that comes in pink, yellow, and blue. The color and taste come mostly from fruits and vegetables, avoiding artificial dyes and flavorings. But, come on, do we really need organic junk food? Cookies, candies, cakes, and chips made with some organic ingredients are still junk food, minus a few toxins.
Reference: *Body & Soul*, "A Sweeter Spin," *Body & Soul*, Sept. 2007, 24(6):26.

We need to buy local, support our local co-ops, and go organic. It's good for the environment and it's good for us.

Organic farmers are speaking out. One of these, Mary-Howell Martens, who with her family organically farms 1,400 acres, testified in the US House of Representatives in 2007. She stressed that organic farmers "have delighted in many, many weed-free, high-yielding fields of organic crops and pastures of healthy, high-producing organic cows, all without pesticides and antibiotics, because organic farming *does* work, it works very well, reliably producing highly productive, high-quality food and feed." She explained that many people don't know much about organic farming and tend to define them by what they *don't* do (such as no pesticides, synthetic fertilizers, antibiotics, GMOs, etc.), which is true. But, what is more important is to define them by what they *do* (diverse crop rotation, soil healthy management, pasture management, intentional biodiversity, cultural weed control, and more). Good organic farming is not simply substituting allowed products for prohibited ones. Rather, it requires that farmers "look upstream" to determine and manage the causes of problems such as weeds and disease, instead of just treating the symptoms. It is about working for a healthy earth as well as healthy people.
Reference: Mary-Howell Martens, "Transitions," *Acres USA*, Sept. 2007: 37(9):14-15.

More and more studies are demonstrating the nutritional superiority of organic produce. In the June 23, 2007 issue of the *Journal of Food and Agricultural Chemistry*, results of a study on tomatoes showed that the level of quercitin, a flavonoid nutrient, increased 79% as a result of long-term organic management. The levels of the flavonoid nutrient kaempferol rose 97%. In addition, the scientists concluded that, the longer a field was managed organically, the bigger the margin of flavonoid levels between organic and conventional plots. In other words, the longer a field was farmed organically, the higher the nutrient content. The longer a field was farmed conventionally, the lower the nutrient content. If you want nutrients, which tomato would you choose?
Reference: "Tomatoes Love Organics," *Acres USA,* Sept. 2007: 37(9):8.

WHAT DO WE DO NOW?

Omega-3 fatty acids used to be quite plentiful in the American diet—in meat, milk products, and eggs from animals raised as Nature intended and from seeds, berries, and green vegetables from the wild or from gardens and farms that used compost, manure, and hands-on attention rather than synthetic fertilizers, toxic pesticides, and huge impersonal machines. We now get only 1/6th of the omega-3s that people got 150 years ago.

"From the perspective of health, the extra effort required to obtain foods that are garden-fresh, sun-ripened, organic, in season, locally grown on rich soils, and grown without body-foreign, poisonous pesticides and artificial fertilizers, is worth making."
Reference Erasmus, Udo, *Fats that Heal, Fats that Kill*, Burnaby BC Canada: Alive Books, 1993: 317.

Chapter Five

WHAT'S IN YOUR MOUTH?

I remember an older woman who came to see the chiropractor I worked with years ago. She became alarmed when she learned that I didn't eat refined sugar. The next time she came to the office she brought some cookies for me, loaded with the white stuff. She said she was afraid that I would get sick if I didn't eat sugar. She was as sweet as the sugar, but, like many people, she only knew what she had eaten all her life and considered this the best way to eat.

Nowadays, I hope, more people know better. Nevertheless, we all tend to enjoy eating the things we are used to eating. Like Mark Twain said, "I'm all for progress; it's change I can't stand." Many people want to eat a healthy diet, but it doesn't translate into actually eating healthy. It's difficult, it requires effort, and it's not as convenient as grabbing a burger on the go. But I find there is another barrier; very often there is confusion about which foods are healthful and which foods are not. I can't tell you how many times people have come to me for a nutritional consultation and claimed that they were already eating a "good" diet, but when we reviewed their eating habits, I usually wanted to moan.

So let's have a quick review. There are *real foods* and there are *nonfoods* (which include what we might call unfoods—they used to be real foods, but were changed into nonfoods or something close to nonfoods). The idea is to eat mostly or all real foods, nutrient-dense foods, things that feed your body. Reduce or eliminate nonfoods, items low or devoid of nutrients and other real food components, items that disrupt or take something from your body, things that expose you to foreign chemicals or toxins, or things that otherwise may please your palate but sabotage your health.

GENERAL DIETARY SUGGESTIONS

It is essential to eat *whole, natural, real foods,* and to avoid the nutritionally impoverished, over-processed, altered, or fake foods. Eat only foods that will spoil and eat them before they do. Get the freshest foods you can and eat them soon. The only way to achieve real health is to eat real food.

You knew that *vegetables* and *fruits* would be at the top of the list as real foods. There are thousands of nutrients and other beneficial ingredients in vegetables and fruits.

Vegetables

Supportive: Fresh vegetables are best, frozen occasionally. Eat raw veggies when you can, such as salads (eat first in your meals if you want to watch your weight), snacks (try soaking carrots, celery, cucumber slices and other veggies in a jar filled with water and a little raw apple cider vinegar—keep cold for snack attacks), in sandwiches, and freshly-made juices. Lightly cook some vegetables; they can be steamed, braised, sautéed, or stewed. Bake others (such potatoes, sweet potatoes, winter squash, and the like). Get organically grown whenever possible. Focus on whatever is in season. Try vegetables you haven't had before. Include leafy greens (not "whites" like iceberg lettuce or French endive or white asparagus).

Non-supportive: Pass on the vegetables in cans; they're cooked to death, often with additives and/or refined sweeteners included. This also applies to canned or bottled juices. The exception is probably canned tomatoes (or tomato sauce or paste) if you must. French fries, ketchup, and sweet pickles do not qualify as vegetables in my opinion, even if government agencies may count them so. They are unfoods. Avoid waxed vegetables if you can; commercially applied wax often contains pesticide residues.

Fruit

Supportive: Again, fresh is best. Eat plenty of it raw, occasionally lightly cooked or frozen. Dried fruits are fine (raisins, figs, dates, apricots, and the like) in moderation, preferably sun-dried. Include fruits in your freshly-made juices. Get organically grown fruit whenever possible, of course, and try to stick to what is in season and grown as close to home as is available.

Non-supportive: Canned fruits are overcooked and usually loaded with refined sweeteners. Stay away from waxed fruit if you can. Avoid irradiated, sprayed, and processed fruits. Don't get dried fruits that are chemically sulfured or sweetened. Don't buy canned or bottled fruit juices; they are usually pasteurized (destroying enzymes and many nutrients) and are highly acidic. Kool Aid is not fruit juice and Fruit Loops are not good sources of fruit. Watch out for items that appear to contain fruit—such as breakfast cereals, fruit drinks, energy bars—but contain only token bits (that are highly processed) or none at all. Some children have told me that real raw fruits, like grapes or strawberries, "don't taste right." They were so used to artificially-flavored grape or strawberry concoctions that the real thing was unrecognizable. Biting into an organically-grown, ripened-on-the-farm peach or cherry could and should send you into bliss.

Vegetables and fruits have been getting a lot of intense study by scientists. They seem to prevent or help just about every health issue and disease around, from macular degeneration to osteoporosis, memory loss to arthritis, insomnia to fluid retention, heart disease to cancer, asthma to diabetes. You name it and they can help. This includes helping you lose weight and feel really good.

Legumes

Supportive: Legumes, beans, and lentils also get good press for all sorts of health benefits such as helping to keep the digestive tract in good order, keeping your mind in good working condition, preventing cancer, and much more. Get 'em young and fresh or dried. Some can be eaten raw, such as sugar snap peas and string beans (try 'em). Others can be cooked fresh such as fava beans, lima beans, and string beans; just don't overcook. Dried beans and lentils need to be soaked to get the germination process going, which disengages the enzyme inhibitors and nutrient-interferers. Soak before cooking (split peas and lentils for two to six hours, most other beans eight to 12 hours, soy 24 hours with water changes every eight hours); strain off water, add fresh water and cook. Any soy products eaten *must* be properly prepared (soaked 24 hours as mentioned) or fermented (as in real fermented soy sauce, tamari, tempeh, or miso). Tofu is a refined food, but because it is fermented, it is tolerable, though not a nutritional bang. Edame is okay if young and fresh. Organically sourced if available. Try different types of legumes like garbanzos, kidney beans, black beans, black-eyed peas, red lentils, and any others you haven't had before.

Non-supportive: Most soy products in the US. Soy is not really the ultimate health food, regardless of the hype. Other beans contain as much and even more of the phytochemicals and nutrients for which soy is lauded. But soy is cheap to grow and process. Asians learned a long time ago that soy must be eaten when it is young and fresh (like edame), otherwise it must be soaked for a long time—longer than other beans (24 hours as mentioned above)—or fermented to be digestible and healthful. If it's not soaked or fermented, there can be problems with nutrient inhibition or interference as well as a few other glitches involving disturbances of your body's chemistry. Most soy products, like veggie burgers, soy milk, soy cheeses, and the like, are made from isolated soy protein, the stuff left over after pressing soybeans for soy oil. Properly prepared (soaked or fermented) soy can be a real food, though not the way to eternal salvation. Isolated soy protein and all the products made from it are unfoods, some are outright nonfoods. Over the years, some of my clients thought a miracle occurred after I suggested they avoid such products. Headaches, fatigue, indigestion, and other symptoms disappeared because most soy products have not been fermented or soaked for a long time.

Most canned beans have not been soaked, though, in a pinch, you may use them. Peanuts are legumes, not nuts. You may think this is a sacrilege, but roasted peanuts, as well as peanut butter, may not be good for you. Many food manufacturers roast the peanuts at high temperatures, creating nasty things in the peanut's oil. There's a huge problem in the US with peanut allergies, yet in other countries, like China, where peanuts are consumed in large amounts, there is hardly any problem at all. Why? Scientists believe it's the high roasting temperatures. In China and in the Southern US, people eat mostly boiled peanuts.

Any beans can cause intestinal gas (flatulence in medical jargon). This is usually due to one or two things: (1) the beans were not soaked and the soaking water replaced with fresh water before cooking, or (2) beans are new to your diet; they are high in fiber and if you're not used to all that good fiber, start with small amounts and gradually eat more (better for you and for those around you).

Nuts and Seeds

Supportive: Nuts and seeds are not just for squirrels and birds. Raw, they are terrific sources of protein, good fats, and minerals. Yes, they contain plenty of fat, but, rather than causing problems, they help many health conditions. Nuts and seeds aid in preventing cardiovascular disease, for one thing, and can help with weight loss, along with a plethora of other ills. Buy them raw in their shells, or, if shelled, make sure the nuts and seeds are really fresh. Chop or grind them, if you please. Make or get raw nut butters, not roasted nut butters. Lightly toast them sometimes. Toss them in salads or stir-fries. Munch for snacks or use as garnishes. Try fresh sesame tahini drizzled on a salad (perhaps mixed with some balsamic vinegar or light miso) or on cooked veggies or in a sandwich. You can make your own version of a nut butter by grinding raw nuts mixed with a little oil or butter.

Non-supportive: Avoid nuts and seeds roasted at high temperatures as well as stale or rancid versions. Some folks find that soaking seeds (like sunflower seeds) for eight or 10 hours makes them much more digestible.

Grains

Supportive: Grains are confusing to some folks. Here's some good advice: look for the word "whole." Like "whole" wheat or rye or quinoa or whatever. "Brown" rice is whole whereas white rice is not. If you see words on a label such as "wheat flour," "semolina flour," or "wheat," it means refined, stripped of at least 70% of their nutrients, their fats (and fat-soluble nutrients such as vitamin E), and most of their fiber. They are unfoods. But they have a long shelf life (good for profits, not for you). Get whole grain breads and other whole grain products. Eat them before they become rancid or moldy. Many whole grains (such as brown rice) are better kept in the refrigerator.

Whole oat groats or steel-cut oats (aka Irish or Scottish oatmeal) are better than rolled oats. Try other whole grains such as millet, barley, quinoa, amaranth, spelt, kamut, teff, and buckwheat. Yes, you can try the exotic ones, which are mostly "new" very old traditional grains. They're good for you and have marvelously different flavors and textures. Sprouted or sourdough bakery products like breads are very good. Whole grain cold breakfast cereals—flakes, puffs, and others—are better than the refined ones, but not nearly as nutritious as grains you cook yourself. Grains are seeds, so they should be soaked or sprouted or fermented (like sourdough) for best nutrient availability. For example, if you want oatmeal in the morning, just put the oats in the pan the night before and soak them along with sufficient water. Next morning, cook (you don't need to change the water). Simple. You want rice for supper? Start soaking in the pan in the morning (or even the night before); in the evening, cook.

Non-supportive: Avoid refined grains and flours as much as you can. Also avoid bleached and "enriched" grain products. Most commercial "whole wheat" and other whole grain flour products may be treated with bleaching chemicals. The now-it-can-go-rancid whole grain flour is processed with toxic chlorine chemicals. The goal is longer shelf life. "Enriched" or "fortified" bakery products should be left on the shelf. Refined grains have had many nutrients natural to the grains removed; manufacturers add back a measly few facsimiles of what was in the grain or add a separated or imitation nutrient that never was in the grain. These chemicals are not the same as the complex nutrient networks in real foods. Actually, "enriched" tells you that a bunch of good stuff has been removed from the grain product and a piddling attempt has been made to put a small number of poor chemical substitutes back in. Unfood and nonfood. And stay away from "instant" cereals; they've been precooked and you cook them again for further depletion.

Meats, Poultry, Wild Game, and Eggs

Supportive: For you meat-eaters, look for meats that come from naturally-raised (drug, hormone, and pesticide-residue-free) animals. Fresh is best, but frozen is okay. Organic please. Pasture-fed (or grass-fed) is the absolute best. This meat has more omega-3 fats, other healthy fats, and other nutrients that are low or missing in commercially-raised animals. Wild game is usually quite good, though the stronger taste may take getting used to. New Zealand lamb is often organically-raised, although it may not say so on the label. Poultry should come from really, truly free-range chickens or ducks or turkeys, birds that always have access to grasses, plants, insects, and other goodies they naturally eat. This diet makes them better for you to eat. Eggs should come from happy, healthy birds; they naturally contain more omega 3s, vitamin A, and other good stuff. Eggs and meats from naturally-raised animals will not harm you or your arteries or any other parts.

Non-supportive: Commercial meats contain residues of pesticides, hormones, and other drugs; the animals are raised in unhealthy, unnatural environments that affect the quality of their meat or eggs or milk. About half of the antibiotics in this country are used on pigs, another reason to get organic pork. Avoid overcooked, processed, commercially-smoked, chemicalized meats such as bacon, ham, luncheon meats, sausages, hot dogs, and so on. Shun them *unless* they have been produced in such a way that nitrates, nitrites, smoking chemicals, refined sugars, synthetic preservatives, and other artificial ingredients have not been used. Don't even consider egg substitutes.

Fish and Seafood

Supportive: Fish and seafood have become controversial subjects. Fish is supposed to be good for you, but it's also polluted these days with mercury, PCBs, dioxins, and many other toxins and poisons. Sometimes farmed fish can be worse because they are fed artificial chemicals in pellets that can contain all sorts of drugs and dyes. However, some aquafarms are raising fish naturally and organically, so there is progress. Know your source. You may need to seek wild sources of smaller ocean fish (fish larger than salmon such as tuna, halibut, swordfish and others contain higher amounts of mercury and other toxins). If you can find out, try to get fish that have not been caught near port cities (the nearer to the shore, the more pollutants).

Non-supportive: Most freshwater fish contain pollutants. As mentioned, turn down the commercially farmed fish and big ocean fish. Pass up the fried fish, processed fish (fish sticks, for example), and most canned seafood. Don't overcook fish and seafood; mostly they require very little cooking time. Check a good cookbook.

Milk and Milk Products

Supportive: Now to the question of milk: not, "got milk?" rather, "which milk?" Certified grade A organic raw milk is the gold standard. Actually, add to that: from pasture-fed animals. In my research and in my experience with people over the years, I have learned that this is definitely the case. Many of you may freak out at the thought of drinking raw milk or using raw milk cheese because we have been told that pasteurized is safer. This is not really true in most cases. Only dirty, contaminated raw milk is harmful. Yet, dirty, contaminated pasteurized milk is also harmful, though it is assumed to be safe because it has been heated. Besides, pasteurization denatures protein, alters fat, destroys enzymes and vitamins, and even changes the milk sugar (lactose) into another form. One of the enzymes destroyed is needed to handle the milk sugar; no doubt this is one reason many people are "lactose intolerant." Did you know that when milk began to be pasteurized, many young children began developing scurvy—an overt deficiency of vitamin C—because the vitamin was no longer in the milk? And did you know that more people become ill from pasteurized milk than from raw milk? It's true. Read Dr. Ron Schmid's book, *The Untold Story of Milk,* if you want the whole story. Even when raw milk products are involved, they usually account for fewer than one percent of the numbers of people affected with illness. And this tiny amount often develops when the milk came from cows in unclean environments. Certified raw milk means that the cleanliness of the cows and their environments are inspected and assured to be sanitary and healthful.

A look at the 22 years from 1922 to 1944—back when many families in rural areas had cows—shows, according to the US Public Health Service, that there were a total of 37,965 cases of all kinds of diseases traced to all types of milk and milk products, both pasteurized and raw. This is an average of 1,726 cases a year. For one year, 1944, there were 1,449 milk-related cases, with only 430 attributed to raw milk. There were 20 deaths, with only one attributed to the consumption of raw milk. Even these days, pasteurized milk products cause far more problems than raw milk. Plus, charges against raw milk frequently lack real proof. Once it is discovered that raw milk was consumed, it is assumed to be the culprit, even if it isn't.

The safest raw milk comes from grass-fed cows. Organic Pastures Dairy in California, for example, is a certified organic, pasture-based raw milk dairy. The cows are kept on fresh green pasture all year. The milk is tested daily, is in compliance with raw milk standards set by the California Department of Food and Agriculture, which also regularly tests the milk. The standards require that raw milk contain less than 15,000 bacteria count per milliliter. The average bacteria count per milliliter since the farm began operations in 2002 is 1,354. That's good clean milk. Besides, the bacteria that develop as clean milk ages are beneficial probiotics, produced by fermentation. For commercial milk, the bacteria allowed before pasteurization (depending on the state) is often 200,000 or there is no limit on the number of bacteria allowed. The bacteria don't disappear after pasteurization—they're simply killed and the residue of dead bacteria are not counted. With age the pasteurized milk putrefies or rots.

If raw milk is "certified," it comes from healthy cows raised in clean conditions and will almost never cause health problems. Pasteurization was initiated because many cows were raised in cities in filth and in very unhealthy conditions. Now that milk is usually pasteurized, all sorts of impurities and contaminants are allowed in the milk (including feces and bugs). It's assumed that, because it is pasteurized, there's no harm. Some of you were raised on farms where you had good, raw milk and you thrived on it. I recall clients over the years, particularly children, who were supposedly "allergic" to milk. When they tried raw milk, not only could they handle it, but they thrived on it. Of course, some people truly do have an intolerance to all cow's milk products and some even to the milk of goats and other animals. Some have problems with just cow's milk and can use raw goat's milk, or they can use raw almond milk, or may not need to use any milk at all. In many cases, a problem in the digestive tract is the reason and this can often be remedied.

Get raw-milk organic cheeses if you want cheese. Yogurt, kefir, sour cream, and cottage cheese may be made from pasteurized milk, but if they have active cultures, they are usually fine. Definitely go for organic milk products (to avoid the growth hormone, drug, and pesticide residues), especially the butter. Remember, toxins accumulate in the fat of animals, so non-organic butter is loaded with them.

Non-supportive: A lot of this was covered above. Pasteurized, homogenized, fortified, chemicalized milk products are not terrific foods. Don't even think about eating processed cheeses (like "American"), skim milk, imitation milk products, dried milk, cream substitutes, or coffee whiteners. Yogurt containing refined sweeteners or frozen yogurts should also be passed up. How about ice cream? No matter how you scoop it, frozen milk or cream is not good-for-you food. But for a very occasional treat, get ice cream that is made from real organic cream and that has evaporated cane juice or honey or pure maple syrup as a sweetener.

Did you know that some commercial ice cream products may contain only a little or no cream at all? And this is important: totally avoid using condensed or evaporated milks; they have been processed beyond the limit of retaining any food value and can contain lots of refined sugars. You don't need that.

Fats and Oils

Supportive: What fats and oils are good to use? Fats that naturally occur in whole foods are good. Also, organic butter. *Unrefined oils.* This means extra-virgin olive oil or any other oil that is labeled "unrefined." "Cold-pressed" or "expeller pressed" do not mean unrefined. The best fats for cooking include butter, ghee, and tropical oils (unrefined palm or coconut oils, for example). These oils are not altered or degraded much when subjected to higher heats (up to 375°F); use these for browning, sautéing, or baking. Butter can burn (the protein part, whey, turns brown), but you can use ghee (butter with the whey removed, called "clarified butter") or you can use both butter and an oil together so the butter will not burn so easily. (Butter and olive oil used together are delicious.) Olive oil, peanut oil, Brazilnut oil, hazelnut oil, almond oil, or sesame oil are fine with medium heat (up to 325°F); use for light sautéing, for instance. Safflower, pumpkin seed, or sunflower oils can deal with only very low heat (up to 212°F); they can be used to make sauces or for light baking, for example. Oils that should not be cooked, but are nevertheless good as condiments or in salad dressings, include flaxseed (can become rancid easily, so be careful), hempseed oil, canola oil, walnut oil, and soy oil.

Nonsupportive: Avoid margarine like the plague—yes, *any* margarine, even the type in your health food store made of organic ingredients. They are all nonfood. Margarine is a partially-hydrogenated fat, otherwise known as a trans fat. Avoid *any* product that contains partially-hydrogenated fat; it's in plenty of processed nonfoods like snack foods and prepared items. Since trans fats are now widely known to be toxic, manufacturers are hustling to find other greasy substitutes. Too often they are just as bad, if not worse. When in doubt, do without.

Avoid refined oils. Lard used to be a wonderful fat for cooking, but unless you have an organic source, don't use it. Don't eat deep fried foods—the fried chicken, fried fish, French fries, chips, donuts, or anything else that is placed in extremely hot (reused over and over again) oil. The fats become highly toxic. Yes, it tastes good and it's crunchy, but there are other ways, such as making oven-baked "fries." Olestra and other artificial fats are not going to really help your health, your arteries, or your waistline. Total nonfoods. Your body knows they are aliens.

Sweeteners

Supportive: Raw honey, evaporated cane juice, and pure maple syrup are good natural sweeteners. Fresh or dried fruits can also be used in recipes for sweetening. Evaporated cane juice such as Rapadura (from Rapunzel) is whole sugar cane juice with only its water removed by a low-heat method. Everything else in the whole cane juice remains. Date sugar is made by drying dates and grinding them into a powder; the crystals contain the same nutrients as dates. Brown rice syrup is a traditional Asian sweetener and fig sugar is made of dried figs. Some dieticians and nutritionists argue that these items are not great sources of nutrients, that they're no different from refined sugars. While it's true that many of them don't contain gobs of nutrients, that is not the point in this particular case. The point is that they do contain food factors that the body uses to process and balance the sweet carbohydrate part. They are not going to disrupt your biochemistry like refined sugars. We're not looking to live on this stuff, just to use a little when sweetening is required. They are real foods. Molasses is the syrup that remains after sugar cane or sugar beets have been processed into refined sugars. The juice is boiled three times: The first time, a light molasses is produced for the mildest and sweetest flavor. The second produces dark molasses, less sweet and more concentrated in flavor. The third boiling makes blackstrap molasses, the darkest, least sweet, and most flavorful. Molasses contains respectable amounts of nutrients like calcium, iron, potassium, magnesium, selenium, and manganese. Yet the boiling destroys or depletes all enzymes and many other ingredients. It can be good to use in cooking in small amounts.

Nonsupportive: Refined sugars are unfoods. Whole sugar cane juice, sugar beets, fruit, or other former foods are refined, stripped of all their natural teammates—water, vitamins, minerals, proteins, fiber, and others—and are often processed and purified with various industrial chemicals. All that's left is the "naked carbohydrate," the sweet part. What's taken away is at least partly the stuff that helps our bodies process the sweet part properly. By eating enough of refined sugars, we can lose nutrients from our own reserves, wreak havoc on our blood sugar metabolism, damage our arteries, acquire cavities, and get fat, to name a few of the problems. You don't get nutrients; you lose them.

Refined sugars appear in items like candy, cake, pies, pastry, breakfast cereals, cookies, soda, ice cream, and the like. They also turn up in things like ketchup, pickles, peanut butter, yogurt, prepared foods, and a zillion other products. Read labels!

Besides the word "sugar," the aliases that you may see on labels include: sucrose, glucose, dextrose, fructose, maltose, corn syrup, high-fructose corn syrup (particularly popular and awful), turbinado sugar, brown sugar, dextrin, maltodextrin, invert sugar, and caramel. Be careful when you see "fruit juice concentrate" because it sometimes means sugar refined from fruit. If the label says "grape juice concentrate," for example, the product should taste like grapes. If it doesn't, you've got a refined sugar extracted from grapes which sounds good, but it isn't.

Agave nectar, prepared traditionally, is made from the sap of a succulent plant native to Mexico. Indigenous peoples of Mexico make it by pouring the agave nectar into a pot and boiling it. They get a very dark, thick liquid with a strong flavor and characteristic smell. It contains inulin, a natural soluble fiber that prevents blood sugar spikes. But now that it's commercially prepared, it is refined and filtered—becoming a sweet syrup—meaning it's no longer the entire nectar, regardless of what the label says and it is subjected to high pressure steam and sometimes to very high temperatures. It may be okay to use once in a while in small amounts, but I wouldn't use it a lot. Much of its goodness has been lost.

How about stevia? It comes from a plant native to Paraguay and is accepted as a safe, low-calorie sweetener in some countries. In the US, stevia used to be sold only as a dietary supplement. Why? Because of some safety concerns. Now, it can be sold as a food (a sweetener). Yet, some researchers still have concerns. In most cases, highly purified and refined extracts are used as stevia sweeteners. There is still not enough information about stevia, particularly its extracts, to endorse its use. Maybe it will turn out to be a good thing. Maybe not.

The annual average consumption of refined sugars in the US is now up to 165 pounds per person. Refined sugars are a well-documented contributing factor to the rise of many serious health problems, including diabetes and obesity.

Artificial sweeteners are *not* any better. They're worse. They can convert beverages into "diet" drinks, for instance, (because they reduce the number of calories) or, to avoid having to use the dreaded "d" word (diet), into "lite" beverages. They're used in chewing gum and other products too. Aspartame (better known as NutraSweet or Equal), Crystal Light, saccharin, sucralose (Splenda), acesulfame-K, maltitol, sorbitol, xylitol (sweeteners ending in "ol" instead of "ose" are sugar alcohols that you can't easily digest), and others are all substances that are *not* found in Nature. They don't seem to control weight. They frequently do have reported side effects (such as nerve damage from consuming lots of aspartame and possibly cancer from saccharin), and they can confuse your body. When you eat something that contains an artificial sweetener, your body assumes sugar is coming, so it gets ready. Sugar doesn't come, but some foreign substance does, leaving your biochemistry in disarray. Long-term use can only cause more disruptions. Between 1980 and 1995, the FDA (Food and Drug Administration) received more than 7,000 complaints from people consuming aspartame including dizziness, headaches, or other unpleasant symptoms. Splenda uses phosgene, a poison gas, in its chlorination process. It's not metabolized (processed in the body) and could be unsafe. Sugar alcohols can have a laxative effect, among other things. All artificial sweeteners are phony. Nonfood.

Condiments
Supportive: Natural herbs and spices. Unrefined sea salt. Raw apple cider vinegar, real wine vinegar, Balsamic vinegar, rice vinegar. Properly fermented miso, tamari, and soy sauce. Natural pickles, olives, mustard. Ketchup and other sauces that do not contain refined sugars or altered fats. All can come into the real food category. Homemade mayonnaise is best since the oil in even organic mayonnaise is heated and refined. It doesn't take long to make your own mayonnaise and it's not difficult. It is so much better.

Nonsupportive: Commercial salt (sodium chloride by itself with chemical additives) and white vinegar are unfoods or nonfoods. Processed mayonnaise, relish, and other condiments that contain refined sugars, altered fats (refined oils, partially-hydrogenated oils), and/or additives (like hydrolyzed protein, MSG, chemical preservatives, artificial flavors...you get the idea) should receive nothing but a cursory glance. A disdainful one.

Beverages
Supportive: What does one drink? Water is the best thing. Water? Just mentioning

this word has brought so many blank, shocked, or incredulous looks from people that I now expect this kind of reaction. Good water actually tastes good and is the best beverage for your body. Natural spring water, tested well water, or properly purified water is the route to take. Most filters and some purifiers do not remove all the harmful chemicals (including fluoride, aluminum, and chlorine) that may be in your tap water. But there are some purifiers that do a thorough job of removing toxins and, unfortunately, may remove some minerals too. Be careful of bottled waters. Some are nothing more than lightly filtered tap water and may be no better (or even worse) than water from your own tap. Additionally, the soft plastic bottles can leach plasticizers that are toxic. Hard plastic or glass bottles which house good, clean spring water are much better. But, to cut back on plastic and expense, find a good filtering or purifying system for your home.

Freshly made vegetable and fruit juices are excellent and will boost your nutrient consumption. Natural herb teas are fine. Green or black tea might be fine occasionally, but tea bushes have an affinity for fluoride, so, with the wide use of artificial fertilizers, there may be more unnatural fluoride in tea than is desirable. Organic sources may be somewhat safer. Coffee (get organic if you can) is okay for most people in limited amounts. If you want decaffeinated coffee, make sure the label says "naturally decaffeinated" to avoid the chemical residues from other methods used to process it.

Wine or beer may be fine, particularly if it is organic and unpasteurized. In moderation, of course. Look for the Mom and Pop breweries and local organic wineries, or, make your own.

Nonsupportive: Soda, juice drinks, latte, and other drinks containing refined sugars, phosphates, chemical additives, and very little if anything resembling real food, should not touch your lips. I have known people who literally had withdrawal symptoms trying to break their particular soda habit. It ain't easy, but it's well worth it.

Will you be able to instantly change your diet to being totally good and healthy? Probably not. We all tend to like what we are used to and change is a struggle. Yet, we weren't born craving unhealthy nonfoods. What dietary habits we formed as children and adolescents greatly influence what we choose to eat as adults. Once those habits are formed (sometimes carved in stone?), our brains and biochemistry can get scrambled enough so that we want those nonfoods; they are the things that taste good to us. White bread tastes good; whole grain bread does not. Ice cream for dessert is yummy; fresh fruit is not sweet enough and is not creamy. French fries may be your vegetable of choice; a salad or steamed broccoli is not even close to being as appealing. You know the drill. We also eat for comfort, as a reward, to compensate for loneliness, depression, anxiety, boredom, or lack of fulfillment. "Junk" food is everywhere we look and easy to obtain; we get lured by smells and sights. These are the barriers.

More than information (even the best information) is required. We need reasons for making changes. Perhaps we have a health problem like arthritis, frequent colds, depression, high blood pressure, chronic fatigue, or something else. Perhaps we are concerned about getting older, being sick, unable to do what we want, being dependent, or looking like a dried-up prune. There may be a history of disease in our families that we want to avoid such as cancer, heart disease, stroke, Parkinson's or Alzheimer's disease. We don't want to pass along our bad habits to our children or grandchildren. These are motivations.

Once you define your motivations, then you can begin to set expectations. You're in a better position to do more for your health than anyone else. First of all, it may be best to take one thing at a time. What do you think you could do for starters? Can you identify any specific barriers that may prevent you from attaining this goal? Do you have confidence that you can reach your goal? For example, you may want to reduce your intake of sweets, but that could be too much to take on. Why not start with soda? Barriers may include your habit of drinking soda while you work, or with your meals, or using it as a substitute for eating other sweets. Strategies may include substituting at first, perhaps drinking naturally-sparkling water with a squeeze of lemon or orange or lime juice and/or eating more naturally-sweet fresh fruit. What is your level of confidence (on a scale from 1 to 10) that you can attain your goal of avoiding soda, perhaps five out of seven days a week? If it's seven or above, then you're on your way.

Other hints as you proceed with reducing or eliminating nonfoods and increasing and including more real foods include using fresh herbs and spices (which resensitize taste buds that have been overwhelmed by refined sugars, altered fats, and the like), focusing on your food (while preparing it and eating it so you'll have more awareness of what and how much you're eating), and creating new recipes.

Generally, try to get as many organic foods as you can. If you can't find organic, get it from a local source (because it's usually fresher and fewer toxins are used). Obtaining foods that are grown or raised locally is a good idea anyway since they will tend to contain more nutrients (they haven't traveled from far away, haven't been harvested before their prime, and haven't been stored very long). Don't cook with very high temperatures. More research is showing that meats and other proteins, grains and other carbohydrates, and fats cooked with high heat produce toxins that can cause health problems such as cancer. Use lower temperatures and, if needed, longer cooking times.

During the earlier years of the 1900s (from the 1920s through the 1970s), many pioneers in nutrition observed the effects of people consuming whole, natural foods and those consuming stripped manufactured nonfoods. Dr. Royal Lee persistently warned against the hazards associated with refined and chemically-adulterated foods that suffered great losses of nutrients. Dr. Weston Price was amazed at the fat-soluble vitamins (such as vitamins A and E) that very healthy, traditional peoples consumed in natural fat-containing foods in amounts that were far greater than what unhealthy, modern peoples consumed in their meddled-with foods. Dr. Francis Pottenger showed the benefits of eating raw foods over cooked foods in his extensive experiments with cats—benefits that extended for generations. Dr. Henry Bieler helped so many people by giving them real natural foods supplying needed nutrients that he had to write a book about it. Dr. Melvin Page stressed the importance of vegetables, especially the green leafy types, as well as getting high quality, properly prepared proteins and unprocessed fats. Such nutritional sages and their words of wisdom were usually dismissed by the scientific community, regsrdless of the incredible health benefits they heralded.

For many years, "scientific" dieticians have subscribed to the notion that "there are no bad foods" (whether Snickers or snack cakes, hot dogs or Hot Pockets) and that anything is fine. You just need to count your calories, avoid as much fat as you can, and get the minimum required nutrients whether they come from foods or are synthetically added to foods. But now, many dieticians and all worthwhile nutritionists know that this is not the way to go. It doesn't work if your goal is wellness. There is a difference between real natural foods and the fabricated, trumped-up, stripped-down excuses for food that make money for manufacturers rather than well-being for consumers. As long as commercial interests have you hooked on nonfoods, they win and you lose. The choice is yours. Wouldn't you rather win better health, more vitality, a positive outlook, and a sparkling appearance by giving your body the authentic, nutrient-dense foods it needs? What's in your mouth?

Keep in your mind a question posed by Claude Fischer, a sociologist with the French National Center for Scientific Research, once asked: "If you are what you eat and you don't know what you're eating, do you know who you are?"

References:

"Beyond the Sugar Bowl: Sweeteners Closer to Mother Nature," *Environmental Nutrition*, June 2007: 30(6), 2.

Colbin, Annemarie, *Food and Healing*, New York: Ballantine Books, 1996.

DeCava, Judith A., *Nutrition News and Views*, "The Whole Food and Nothing but the Food," May/June 2006: 10(3).1-6; "Let Food Be Your Medicine," Mar./Apr. 2002: 6(2),1-6; "Non-food Versus Real Food," Mar./Apr. 2005: 9(2), 1-6 for more information and numerous references.

Eating Well, Feb./Mar. 2005: 3(3), 8.

Lark, Susan M., "Beat Unhealthy Food Cravings and Addictions," *Women's Wellness Today*, Oct. 2008: 15(10), 1-6.

Nagel, Rami, "Agave: Nectar of the Gods?," *Wise Traditions*, Summer 2008: 9 (2), 46-51.

Nestle, Marion, *What to Eat*, New York: North Point Press, 2006.

"Resisting Sweet Temptation," *Ode*, June 2007: 5(5), 69.

Robinson, Jo, *Pasture Perfect*, Vashon, WA: Vashon Island Press, 2004.

Shardt, David, "Stevia: Sweet...but How Safe?." *Nutrition Action Healthletter*, Oct.2008: 35(8), 9.

Schmid, Ron, *The Untold Story of Milk*, Washington, DC: New Trends Publishing, Inc., 2003.

Schmid, Ronald F., *Traditional Foods Are Your Best Medicine*, Rochester, VT: Healing Arts Press, 1997.

"We Want to Eat Right, but...," *Tufts University Health & Nutrition Letter*, June 2007: 25(4), 3.

What's in a Grain of Wheat?

Endosperm
The biggest starchy carbohydrate part of the wheat kernel that contains a bit of protein and tiny amounts of nutrients. This is the part of the wheat seed that feeds the little growing plant and essentially the only part left when wheat is refined into white flour.

Bran
The outer layers that contain most of the fiber as well as some B vitamins, minerals, protein and antioxidants (which protect nutrients from breaking down too quickly).

Wheat Germ
This is the inner nugget, the nutrient-rich part that is full of B vitamins, vita min E, good fats, minerals, and some proteins

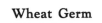

WHAT'S IN YOUR MOUTH?

In the United States, wheat is usually eaten in its least nutritional form—stripped of the nutrient-dense parts (germ and bran layers) and smashed into a fine, starchy powder known as white flour. It is usually bleached (for shelf life), treated with conditioners, preservatives, and other chemicals, then "fortified" with a measly few imitation vitamins and nonfood minerals. Wheat that has been manipulated this way is no longer a real food.

Whole wheat—the real deal—is rich in vitamin E complex, B vitamins (such as B_6 and folate), calcium, magnesium, potassium, zinc, copper, manganese, chromium, and fiber. Vitamin B_4, a nutrient ignored by the scientific community, benefits the function of and nurtures the heart.

Many of the nutrients support the nervous system, aiding mood and focus and our ability to deal with stress. Whole wheat supports organs and glands, blood vessels and hormones, muscles and bones, digestion and weight balance, blood sugar balance and longevity, repair and healing.

When grains are refined, they lose a substantial part of their nutritional value. Here are some of the approximate losses:

Nutrient	Percentage of Loss	Nutrient	Percentage of Loss
Fiber	85	Iron	70 to 76
Thiamine (B_1)	75 to 97	Magnesium	80 to 85
Riboflavin (B_2)	65 t0 80	Potassium	77 to 80
Niacinamide (B_3)	75 to 80	Sodium	78
Pyridoxine (B_6)	72 to 94	Zinc	72 to 85
Pantothenic Acid (B_5)	50 to 57	Copper	68 to 80
Folate (folic acid)	75	Manganese	86 to 90
Biotin	75	Calcium	50-60
Choline	50%	Molybdenum	48
Vitamin E	70 to 88	Phosphorous	71
Selenium	25	Essential fatty acids	70
Cobalt	89	Protein	25 or more

FOOD FOR THOUGHT or should I say,
THOUGHTS FOR FOOD?

Miriam E. Nelson, PhD and Alice H. Lichtenstein, DSc of Tufts University advocate "keeping the emphasis on the whole foods" available in markets, rather than on "the boxed, bagged, canned and other packaged goods lining all the center aisles." Eileen Kennedy, DSc, RD, dean of Tufts Freidman School, says to look for foods that are "nutrient dense." Choose a potato instead of potato chips, or a banana instead of a soda. Opt for a plate loaded with vegetables and skip the dinner roll made of refined flour. Ignore the cake and go for the fresh fruit. Choosing foods based on nutrient density means "choosing foods based on quality." Don't you deserve it?
Reference: "Smarter—and Healthier—Supermarket Shopping Made Simple," *Tufts University Health & Nutrition Letter*, Sept. 2006: 24(7),4-5.

If you feel overwhelmed or ready to run when you walk into your local supermarket, you are normal. There are thousands of products, packaging that touts ever-changing health claims, and tempting displays. Stores are designed to make you do a lot of impulse buying. To arm yourself, first prioritize by jotting down what you actually need and stay on track with it. Don't go to the store at its busiest times or when you're hungry. Set a time limit. Use a basket or smaller cart rather than a big shopping cart which you will tend to fill up. Stick with your health goals and values by keeping your priorities in mind so you will stay focused. Remember, people will often choose what is most visible. Research shows that we each make over 200 food-related decisions every day, though we may only be aware of about 30 of them. Read labels. Spend most of your time in the perimeter of the grocery store where most of the fresh, whole foods reside. "Conscious eating is about knowledge," notes professional chef and nutrition adviser Stephanie Bryn Sacks, MS. Are you armed and ready?
Reference: Goldman, Sharon M., "Buy Better Groceries," *Body & Soul*,Jan./Feb. 2007: 24(1), 46-51.

The party line some dietitians adhere to is "there are no bad foods." But increasing numbers of dietitians are realizing that it is critical that consumers recognize that there are foods they should eat less of and some they should avoid. Strange; we underrated nutritionists have been saying that for many years.

More than half of North Americans are aware of what they should be eating, but most don't follow it. For the most part, consumers aren't willing to trade convenience for health or other benefits. "Products cannot be healthful at the expense of convenience or they will not be successful." Am I weird because I not only value my health, but I enjoy real, healthful foods? What's so difficult about grabbing an apple, throwing together a salad, or making a stir fry? Are you willing to sacrifice your health for the sake of convenience? Should good food be what you wished you ate but didn't bother to? It's *your* health, *your* appearance, and the length of *your* life.

WHAT'S IN YOUR MOUTH?

Reference: "We Want To Eat Right, But…," *Tufts University Health & Nutrition Letter*, June 2007: 25(4), 3.

The word "refined" in the food world means that unwanted materials are removed. For the most part, the parts that are removed are those unwanted by food manufacturers, not by your body. Refined foods are often over-processed, complete with additives and preservatives to allow for increased shelf life, attractiveness, mouth-feel, flavor, packaging, and shipping.

Whenever a refined- and over-processed-foods diet has been introduced to a traditional culture anywhere in the world, a general degradation of the people's health follows, usually within one generation. From tooth decay to diabetes, arthritis to ulcers, cardiovascular disease to cancer, numerous degenerative conditions, immune-compromising illnesses, gland and hormone disruptions, nerve diseases, and other health problems develop. Soon they match the condition of people in industrialized societies.

Dr Weston A. Price, a dentist and researcher, observed and described this phenomenon back in the 1930s and 1940s. He studied native cultures eating modern refined and processed diets and compared them to similar groups who were still eating their traditional, natural diet. The differences were amazing and indisputable.

Reference: Price, Weston A., *Nutrition and Physical Degeneration: A Comparison of Primitive Diets and Their Effects*, La Mesa: Price-Pottenger Nutrition Foundation, original 1948, current 1998.

Of course, the term "whole food" is relative. The hull of a grain kernel is an outer shell that is hard, tough and inedible. It must be removed to use the grain. The cane of the sugarcane is too tough to eat, so the juice inside is used. Refined sugar is virtually all sucrose. The whole liquid from the sugar cane is only 10 to 18% sucrose. It also contains valuable minerals, organic acids, pectin, and gums which aid your body in using the sucrose sugar properly.

Seeds, nuts, grains, beans, and fruits used for oil are, obviously, no longer "whole," but the body can still use the oils as valuable food if they are carefully extracted or pressed and properly handled. The shells of nuts and seeds have to be removed. Some vegetables and fruits either have to be peeled or we don't eat the peel (such as winter squash or avocados). We don't eat a whole steer or cow, but parts of it. We remove the head and feet and guts of poultry, we scale fish, soak beans, chop and cut foods, and cook some of them. All of these procedures can be called "processing."

But when we use the term "processed food," we're essentially referring to foods that have been *over-processed*—subjected to procedures that go beyond what is necessary to make them edible—and/or inflicted with chemical additives. Such items have been altered from their original essence and contaminated with substances foreign to their nature and toxic to ours.

Reference: Kilham, Chris, *The Whole Food Bible*, Rochester: Healing Arts Press, 1997: 9, 23-30, 98-110

Whole foods, then, are minimally refined when necessary so we can eat them. They keep maximum nutritional value. Whole foods provide, not only nutrients in natural proportion to each other, but the nutrients are all bound together—integrated—in a network that makes the whole far more healthful than any separated parts.

So you don't have to eat banana skins, walnut shells, or fish bones to be eating "whole" foods. Still, some parts of foods considered inedible can be transformed into appetizing, nourishing morsels. For example, bones (along with aromatic vegetables, seasonings and water) make wonderful, nutritious broths and stocks. Watermelon rinds can be pickled. Organic orange or lemon rinds can be grated.

Fruits and Vegetables:

Despite all the nagging from nutritionists like me as well as health journals and the government, most Americans are still not eating enough fruits and vegetables. In 2005, 32.6% of the US adult population consumed fruit two or more times a day, and 27.2% ate vegetables three or more times a day. The number one vegetable consumed is French fries. When students in grades 9 through 12 were asked about eating fruits and vegetables five or more times a day, only 16.9% did so.

Reference: "Americans Falling Short of Fruit, Veggie Goals," *Nutrition Week*, 26 Mar. 2007: 37(6), 3, and "Tracking Health-related Behaviors at the School Level," 12 Mar. 2007, 37(5), 8.

The avocado is a fruit. The fat in avocados may help your body's ability to absorb certain nutrients. One such nutrient is lycopene, which might assist in preventing heart disease and prostate cancer. Others include carotenes like beta-carotene, zeaxanthin, and lutein, which may reduce the risk of various cancers and eye diseases. Avocados are rich in fiber, potassium (more than bananas), folate, niacinamide, carotenes to make vitamin A, vitamin C, and phytosterols (stuff that lowers cholesterol). They even have magnesium, vitamins E and K, and a nice amount of glutathione (which helps detoxification). I like them in salads or in salad dressings.

How many of you are old enough to remember the grapefruit diet? Well, a recent study involving obese (really overweight) people showed that grapefruit consumption was indeed associated with weight loss. Of course, I think most any fresh fruits and vegetables will help.

Reference: Fujioka, K., F. Greenway, et al, "The Effects of Grapefruit on Weight and Insulin Resistance: Relationship to the Metabolic Syndrome," *Journal of Medicinal Food*, 2006: 9(1), 49-54.

Are sprouts the ultimate health food? Or are they toxic? Evidently, sprouts of legumes (alfalfa, clover, mung beans, lentils, garbanzos, and the like) develop toxins at a certain stage of growth. These toxins are broken down if you cook the sprouts lightly in water. Alfalfa sprouts contain canavanine, a toxin that can insult the immune system, but cooking turns these sprouts into mush. Other sprouts such as sunflower, radish, and buckwheat are very good, loaded with nutrients and enzymes. Eat them raw.

Can you really get a nutrient bang from chomping a salad? Yes. Salad-eaters were found to have consistently higher levels of many nutrients in their bloodstreams.
Reference: "Greens Are Great, Researchers Say," *Nutrition Week*, 11 Sept. 2006: 37(18), 6.

Eat your greens and eat a variety. Spinach, chard, kale, romaine lettuce, beet greens, arugula, broccoli rabe, and other greens are packed full of important nutrients, including carotenes (like beta-carotene), vitamin K (recently shown to help maintain strong bones), magnesium (which most North Americans are deficient in), and much more. Leafy greens are incredibly high in lutein and zeaxanthin which, among other things, may prevent macular degeneration. These two carotenes are the only ones that accumulate in the lens of the eye, and are most concentrated in the macula (of the retina). Eating watercress daily lowered DNA damage (an indicator of cancer risk) to white blood cells in healthy adults. Dandelion greens rank among the top four green vegetables for overall nutritional value. These greens offer more beta-carotene than carrots, and more iron and calcium than spinach. They're also rich in vitamins C and D, magnesium, phosphorus, vitamin B_1, B_2, and potassium. Would it help if you thought of green leaves as one form of Nature's money? The payoff is tremendous.
References: Barker, Elizabeth, "Wonders of Watercress," *Body & Soul*, July/Aug. 2007: 24(5), 32. [4]
Campbell, Adam, *Men's Health*, June 2007: 50.
Castleman, Michael, "Bitter Treat," *Natural Health*, Apr. 2007: 37(4), 104.
Liebman, Bonnie, "The Greens Party," *Nutrition Action Healthletter*, July/Aug. 2007: 34(6), 10-11.
Roufos, Anna "Eat Your Greens!," *Eating Well*, Dec. 2006: 5(6), 41.

Beets have been used for centuries as a remedy for many ailments, from constipation to blood-related problems. The beet root contains pigments that help your body counteract toxins, including some that are potentially cancer-causing. Yes, beet roots contain iron as well as potassium and folate. The greens are rich in potassium, folate, carotenes, and vitamin K. Root and leaf are excellent support to the liver for proper function and excretion of bile. I have used whole beets many times in programs for detoxification or cleansing. Our livers love them.
Reference: Redmond, Cheryl, "Power Foods: Beets," *Body & Soul*, July/Aug. 2007: 24 (5), 49-50.

Studies show that celery will lower blood pressure. This puts scientists into a quandary. Because celery has a high-sodium reputation, they tell patients to avoid celery.

However, celery is higher in potassium (known to lower blood pressure) than sodium. Natural, real foods won't cause the imbalances that tampered-with foods may cause. Refined sodium-chloride (table salt) in excess may, and only in some people, lead to higher blood pressure. Yet, even in those folks who react to the salt, the addition of potassium-rich real foods will usually alleviate the blood pressure conundrums.

I remember one older Asian gentleman who developed high blood pressure. His doctor recommended medication, but instead, he decided to eat celery every day, a therapy from his homeland. His blood pressure came down to normal. His doctor's mouth dropped open for a short time. Then, the doctor advised him to stop eating celery because it was high in sodium and might increase his blood pressure, yet the celery had already lowered the man's blood pressure.

Reference: "Celery Deceptively Rich in Phytonutrients," *Environmental Nutrition*, Dec. 2006: 29(12), 7.

Chiles are not related to the pungent berries of the black pepper plant. It was Christopher Columbus who confused them. Yet chiles—from hot habaneros to sweet bells, from cayenne to paprika—are still called "peppers." Capsaicin, a compound in hot chiles, increases the body's metabolic rate (causing you to burn more calories) and may stimulate brain chemicals that help us feel less hungry. So, if you like it hot, indulge.

Reference: "Chile Peppers," *Eating Well*, Jan./Feb. 2007: 6(1), 88.

Red, yellow, and orange bell peppers have more vitamin C than green bells. A 3.5-ounce green pepper has about 80 milligrams of vitamin C, twice as much (ounce for ounce) as an orange. A red pepper has about 125 milligrams in 3.5 ounces and a yellow pepper has about 185 milligrams. Green peppers contain carotenes (like beta-carotene) which increase as peppers mature and turn red or yellow. A red pepper has eight times as much beta-carotene as a green one. Peppers are also a good source of potassium.

Reference: "Peter Piper's Pick," *UC Berkeley Wellness Letter*, July 2007: 23(10), 7.

Artichokes, if unpicked, will blossom into gorgeous purple flowers. What we eat are the buds. Artichokes do wonders for your heart, liver, and sweet tooth. They soothe digestive disturbances such as nausea, pain, and bloating. The flavonoid silymarin in them boosts liver function, helping it to regenerate, scavenge and deal with toxins, and promote bile production which helps fat digestion. Artichokes stimulate sweet receptors so anything you eat after them will taste sweet, even water.

Reference: Black, Jane, "Power Foods: Artichokes," *Body & Soul*, Apr./May 2007: 24(3), 53-54.

Cooked asparagus and its watery juices can help dissolve uric acid deposits, such as gout, in the extremities. It also helps you urinate if you are having trouble doing so.

Reference: Heinerman, John, *Heinerman's New Encyclopedia of Fruits & Vegetables*, West Nyack, NY: Parker Publishing Company, 1995:14-15.

The humble cabbage may help prevent cancer, lower serum cholesterol, increase elimination, fight yeast infections (taken internally or used as a vaginal douche or both), help heal stomach or intestinal ulcers, and assist in protecting you from harmful effects of radiation.

Reference: Heinerman, John, *Heinerman's New Encyclopedia of Fruits & Vegetables*, West Nyack, NY: Parker Publishing Company, 1995: 74-77.]

Processed potatoes, from dehydrated flakes and frozen fries to mashed puffs and *Tater Tots*, may be convenient, but all that processing either destroys or removes nutrients like vitamin C, potassium, and fiber, while adding questionable or downright toxic fats and lots of salt.

Reference: "Packages Potatoes: More Convenient, Less Nutritious," *Environmental Nutrition*, June 2007: 30(6), 5.

Many recipes call for the removal of the peel and seeds of tomatoes. Don't do it if you want to maximize the amount of nutrients you can get from your tomatoes. Eat and cook them in their natural state, with seeds and peel.

Reference: "Food as Preventive: Symposium Highlights Hidden Health Power of Foods," *Environmental Nutrition*, Dec. 2006: 29(12), 3.

Researchers have found that sea vegetables, like kelp and other seaweeds, are loaded with components that are believed to protect against cancer, heart disease, the common cold, osteoporosis, and other ills, as well as cleanse the digestive tract. Yes, they are a good way to get iodine for your thyroid gland, and they're also full of carotenes, B vitamins, and vitamin K as well as calcium, magnesium, iron, phosphorus, manganese, and zinc. Alginic acid, abundant in seaweed, can bind with toxic heavy metals (like mercury, barium, cadmium, lead, and radioactive strontium), making them indigestible and easily eliminated.

Reference: Gusman, Jill, "Sea Sides," *Natural Health*, Sept. 2007: 37(8), 43-49.

Drinking fruit and vegetable juices at least three times a week might reduce the risk of Alzheimer's disease by as much as 75%. Juices may also help protect us from cardiovascular disease and cancer. There's much more than fiber in fruits and vegetables. Remember, freshly-made juices are best. Bottled, canned, or boxed are greatly inferior.

Reference: "Research Roundup," *Environmental Nutrition*, Nov. 2006: 29(11), 8. and Ruxton, C.H., E.J. Gardner, et al, "Can Pure Fruit and Vegetable Juices Protect Against Cancer and Cardiovascular Disease Too? A Review of the Evidence," *Journal of Food, Science, and Nutrition*, 2006: 57(3-4), 249-272.

A group of people was asked to eat a little over half a pound of cherries every day for a month. A blood marker of inflammation, C-reactive protein, decreased by 25%. Other signs of inflammation also decreased during the study and for a good month following the study. Did blood sugar levels spike up from all this fruit? No, they didn't. Fasting blood sugar and insulin levels were unchanged. Triglycerides (a sign of stored sugars) were not affected either. Cherries are famous for helping people with gout.

Reference: Fuchs, Nan Kathryn, "Are Cherries Too Sweet To Eat Every Day?," *Women's Health Letter*, Sept. 2002: 12(9), 4-5.

I'll bet you keep watermelon in the fridge. Yet storing fruits, tomatoes, and some vegetables at room temperature makes them taste better than when they are stored in the refrigerator. There's more. Storage of watermelons at room temperature increases their content of carotenes like lycopene and beta-carotene. The key is to get fruits and vegetables fresh and eat them as soon as you can to avoid spoilage from storing them a long time.

Reference: Perkins-Veazie, P., and J.K. Collins, "Carotenoid Changes of Intact Watermelons After Storage," *Journal of Agriculture and Food Chemistry*, 2006: 54:5868-5874.

Speaking of watermelon, it's also an excellent source of the amino acid citrulline. Our bodies use citrulline to make another amino acid, arginine, which plays a key role in cell division, wound healing, and the removal of ammonia from the body. Arginine is used in the body to make nitric oxide, a signaling molecule that helps regulate blood pressure, improve healthy circulation, and even boost male sexual function. Only a few foods contain high levels of citrulline.

Reference: "Watermelon Serves Up Medically Important Amino Acid," ARS News Service, USDA, newsservice@ars.usda.gov, 21 Mar. 2007.

Raspberries are little nuggets of nutrients like vitamin C and manganese (a trace mineral important to bones and ligaments). They are one of only a few foods that contain substantial ellagic acid, a phytonutrient that has potential cancer-protective abilities. Black raspberries have more ellagic acid and more anthocyanins (another phytonutrient) than the red ones.

Reference: "Red or Black, Raspberries Ripe With Phytonutrients," *Environmental Nutrition*, June 2007: 30(6), 7.

"An apple a day keeps the doctor away." There are many reasons this is so. But this old rhyme was originally a polite way of explaining that apples are a good preventive of both constipation and diarrhea. To combat diarrhea, grate an apple and let it stand at room temperature for several hours until it has darkened quite a bit; then eat. The oxidized pectin in the apple will help acute diarrhea such as "Montezuma's Revenge," the bane of tourists. By the way, the seeds in apple cores contain amygdalin, a naturally occurring cyanide/sugar compound that degrades into hydrogen cyanide. Yup, it's a toxin. Swallowing an apple seed or two won't poison you, though eating a lot of apple seeds could be a problem. It's interesting that folks in Peru and other South American countries always eat some seeds when eating an apple since they are a remedy for intestinal parasites.

Reference: Heinerman, John, *Heinerman's New Encyclopedia of Fruits & Vegetables*, West Nyack, NY: Parker Publishing Company, 1995:3-5.

There are more than a thousand kinds of mangos. These fruits each contain 20 times more vitamin A (as carotenes) than an orange.
Reference: "A Guide To Tropical Fruits," *Natural Health*, June 2007: 37(6), 68.

Pomegranates and their juice have received plenty of publicity lately. For one, pomegranates may help men live longer after treatment for prostate cancer. Drinking an 8-ounce glass of the juice slowed the rate at which patients' rising prostate-specific antigen (PSA) levels doubled (from an average of 15 months to 54 months) indicating the progression of their disease slowed down quite a bit. The next step is to see if it helps protect men from developing prostate cancer in the first place. However, as is true with all foods, there are variations in response to pomegranate juice, depending on the individual.
Reference: "Pomegranate Power," *Vegetarian Times*, Oct. 2006: Vol.344:14, and Seeram, Navindra P., Susanne M. Henning, et al, "Pomegranate Juice Ellagitannin Metabolites Are present in Human Plasma and Some Persist in Urine For Up to 48 Hours," *Journal of Nutrition*, Oct. 2006: 136(10), 2481-1485.

Legumes:
"I've been working with beans for 28 years," says Dr. George Hosfield, "and you can't find a better plant food for its proteins, energy, zinc, iron, folic acid and fiber." North Americans average about 150 pounds of refined sugars per year, but less than eight pounds of beans. However, North Americans eat more than 700 million pounds of peanut butter every year.
References: "The Color of Beans," *Eating Well*, Spring 2004: 2(4), 17, and "Did You Know?," *Health & Healing*, Nov. 2005: 15(11), 5.

Soy has been praised as one of the best foods in the world, and scorned as one of the worst foods in the world. Which is it? Neither and both. Soy products are cheap to make because most are made from what is left-over after soy oil has been squeezed out to make refined oils and trans fats. Global production of soybeans increased from 30 million tons in 1965 to 270 million tons in 2005. But soybeans, more than other beans, contain enzyme inhibitors and nutrient inhibitors that are good for the bean to preserve its goodies until it is germinated, but bad for us as its eaters. Asians learned a long time ago that, to use the soybean as a food, it must be soaked for a long time (24 hours, with 8-hour intervals of dumping and replacing the water) or, even better, fermented. This makes it healthier and digestible.

Many studies that find beneficial effects from soy come from Japan or China, or involve Asian Americans, all who use mostly fermented versions. Unfermented or unsoaked soy, what most Americans eat, can cause allergies, intolerances, thyroid stress (if getting inadequate iodine), and interference with nutrient uptake. We've heard so many good things about soy, but, as Leena Hilakivi-Clarke, PhD, explains: "Many condition-specific claims, however, seem to be inflated, misinterpreted, or just not based on sound scientific studies." Soy is not living up to its pumped-up reputation. In fact, other beans contain more isoflavones and other components for which soy has been praised. If you want soy, use real fermented soy sauce (traditional shoyu or tamari), miso, tempeh, natto, and a little tofu (traditionally made, not 'silken'). They're fermented.

References: Barr, Susan Learner, "The Truth About Soy," *Shape*, June 2007:198.

Daniel, Kaayla T., "Soy: Is It Cancer On a Plate?," *What Doctors Don't Tell You*, Nov.2005: 16(8), 7-10.

Hardy, Mary, "Thyroid Function and Soy: The Good, the Bad and the Not-So-Ugly!," *Alternative Therapies in Women's Health*, Mar. 2005: 7(3), 21-24.

Klotter, Jule, "Soy Questions from Britain," *Townsend Letter*, Feb./Mar. 2007: 31.

Besides the boost of fiber and phytonutrients; besides the B vitamins and acytlcholine for your brain and nerves; besides the protein, iron, calcium, zinc, potassium, molybdenum, and other nutrients, beans may help you remove toxins from your intestines, prevent constipation, help reduce your risk of heart disease and certain cancers, and help control your weight as well as your blood sugar. So it's okay to be full of beans. Just make sure you soak them for eight hours or so, discard the soak water, replace with fresh water, and cook. Or begin the fermentation process by adding a little whey or lemon juice in the soaking water. Either way, you won't experience the dreaded flatulence (intestinal gas) and you'll get a lot more absorbable nutrients.

References: "Beans: New Diet Food," *Environmental Nutrition*, June 2006: 29(6), 3.

"Gasless Beans," *Acres USA*, Aug. 2007: 38(8), 73.

Kelly, Karen, "The Bean Scene," *Natural Health*, Dec./Jan. 2007: 37(1), 35-40.

Rogers, Sherry A., "Make Sure You're Full of Beans," Jan. 2005: 6.

UC Berkeley Wellness Letter, Jan. 2006: 22(4), 2-3.

Grains:

Whole grains, three to four servings a day, reduced the risk for periodontitis, the leading cause of tooth loss in adults.

Reference: Merchant, Anwar T., "Whole-Grain and Fiber Intakes and Periodontitis Risk in Men," *American Journal of Clinical Nutrition* June 2006: 83(6), 1395-1400.

Whole-grain products contain all the components of the kernel—the bran, (outer shell), germ (seed), and the soft endosperm. The bran and germ contain most of the fiber, B vitamins, vitamin E, iron, zinc, and other nutrients, plus phytonutrients. Refining grains removes the bran and germ, and thus most of the nutrients and fiber. "Enriched" flour means a few synthetic vitamins and/or non-food minerals have been added to the refined fluff, but these don't even come close to replacing what was lost. Besides, these paltry additions are poor imitations. Some refined grain products have added fiber (from bran, inulin, or guar gum, for instance), but they still lack the nutrients of whole grains. The food package has been broken!

Technically, amaranth, buckwheat, quinoa, and wild rice are not really grains. They don't belong to the grass family. But their nutritional profile is similar, so most experts place them in the same category.

Amaranth is high in protein, gluten-free, and contains as much calcium as milk. The seed of a tall shrub with beautiful magenta flowers, amaranth contains more protein than other grains. And it is higher in calcium, magnesium, and potassium than other grains— half a cup contains 149 milligrams of calcium, the same amount in half a cup of milk. The oil in amaranth is fairly high in linolenic acid, an omega-3 fat, as well as vitamin E complex. Be adventurous and try foods like this if you haven't done so already.

Reference: Fuchs, Nan Kathryn, "Add This Nutrient-Rich Grain to Your Heart-Healthy Diet," *Women's Health Letter*, June 2007: 13(6), 1-2.

In various large studies, people who ate more whole grains had a lower risk of cardio-vascular disease (by about 20%) than those who ate few or no whole grains. Whole grains also improve insulin sensitivity and may help ward off type 2 diabetes (by 23 to 33%). It's also been found that women who ate more whole grains gained less weight over time. And, whole grain consumption is a strong predictor of decreased risk for certain types of cancer. Furthermore, eating whole grains can reduce the risk of dying from inflammatory diseases such as Crohn's disease, emphysema, and chronic obstructive pulmonary disease (COPD). Researchers don't exactly know why whole grains are so good for you. Could it be because they are real whole foods containing a huge bunch of synergistic ingredients?

References: Jacobs, David R., Jr., Lene Frost Andersen, and Rune Blomhoff, "Whole-Grain Consumption is Associated With a Reduced Risk of Noncardiovascular, Noncancer Death Attributed to Inflammatory Diseases in The Iowa Women's Health Study," *American Journal of Clinical Nutrition*, June 2007: 85(6), 1606-1614.

Mellen, Philip B., Angela D. Liese, et al, "Whole-Grain Intake and Carotid Artery Atherosclerosis in a Multiethnic Cohort: The Insulin Resistance Atherosclerosis Study," *American Journal of Clinical Nutrition*, June 2007: 85(6), 1495-1502.

Riccardi, Victoria Abbott, "Old Faithfuls," *Natural Health*, Nov. 2006: 36(10), 39-45.

"Wellness Facts," *UC Berkeley Wellness Letter*, Aug. 2007: 23(11), 1.

Science is finding that eating fiber by itself is not as beneficial as eating fiber consumed as a whole grain. The benefits of whole grains come from what Philip B. Mellen, MD and Frank B. Hu, MD, PhD, call whole grains' "unique constellation of constituents." It's the whole package containing all the fiber, vitamins, minerals, lignans, phenolic compounds, phytochemicals, and other goodies, all refined away along with the germ and bran. Break the package and you destroy the intricate connections. Think of this the next time you reach for bran muffins or bran cereals that simply toss some bran in with refined flour. It's a broken package with missing parts.

Reference: "Five New Reasons to Get Whole Grains," *Tufts University Health & Nutrition Letter*, Aug. 2007: 25(6), 1-2.

An organically-grown or organically-raised food might escape a lot of toxic contamination. Yet it can still be refined. This means the removal of nutrient-dense, fiber-rich, or otherwise valuable portions. For example, whole grain wheat berries can be stripped of their germ and bran, eliminating from 50% to 90% of their various nutrients as well as most of the fiber. "Organic unbleached flour" is refined, not whole wheat. It's better than nonorganic unbleached flour and much better than synthetically-enriched bleached flour. But the narrowed nourishment and loss or wholeness of organic refined flour can easily be avoided by the use of organic *whole* wheat products.

Unless the word "whole" precedes the grain name for wheat, oats, corn, rye, and barley, you can't be sure you're getting the entire intact grain. Even if the word "whole" does not appear on labels before the words brown or wild rice, buckwheat, triticale, bulgur, millet, quinoa, amaranth, and sorghum, you may nevertheless be getting whole grains.

Have you ever tried preparing whole wheat berries—the whole, unprocessed kernels? They take a while to cook (soak first for several hours, then cook for about an hour), but they are yummy, chewy, and chock-full of B vitamins, iron, magnesium, zinc, vitamin E, and fiber. Use them like rice. Did you know that 20% of the world's food calories are supplied by wheat? Unfortunately, most of it has been refined.

Now that whole grains have received a 'thumbs up' from scientists, an amazing array of packaged goods are showing up with "whole grains" on their labels. Multigrain Tostitos have "Four Wholesome Grains," but a one-ounce serving (8 chips) contain more of refined sugar (1 gram) than it does any of those four grains (oat, buckwheat, and whole wheat flour, toasted corn germ). Nabisco Wheat Thins Multi-Grain Toasted Chips are "made with Whole Grain—5 g per serving"—but they consist mostly of refined white flour. The whole grains make up only about a quarter of the grain in a one-ounce (12 chips) serving. The Flat Earth Garlic & Herb Field Baked Veggie Crisps ad says: "½ Serving of Real Vegetables in Every Ounce," but they are mostly refined rice flour and dried potato flakes (the "real vegetable") with a smattering of pumpkin, onion, and tomato paste. Selling tactics are clever and they work. Sounds healthful, but they're nevertheless nonfoods. All chips contain fats heated at high temperatures, not only making altered, toxic fats, but probably creating toxin-containing carbohydrates as well. "Whole grain" on a label doesn't mean the item is a healthy choice.

When bread is toasted, a chemical process takes place that caramelizes the surface sugars and proteins, turning the surface brown. The sugar becomes an indigestible fiber and the protein loses its nutritional value.
Reference: Bader, Myles H., *2001 Food Secrets Revealed*, Las Vegas: Northstar Publishing, 1997: 148.

Fats:
Manufacturers of chips, French fries, and donuts re-use vegetable oils. FFAs (free fatty acids) concentrate in the oil, so to solve this problem the oils are chemically treated. These oils are so bad that biodiesel manufacturers won't use them, but we're supposed to *eat* the chips or fries? One donut shop offered its used oil for free for biodiesel use—a 55-gallon drum once every six months. Have you ever seen the vast amount of oil in the vats used to fry donuts? Yet they dispose of only 55 gallons every six months. It means the oil is used over and over. This has my stomach turning. One closed-down donut shop asked

for a barrel of used vegetable oil to be picked up from its parking lot because it was leaking and causing *environmental damage*. The oil was so thick and sludgy that it clogged the pump used to try to drain the oil. It had an unpleasant smell and was not usable as an ingredient for fuel. Scientific information, such as the carcinogen content of such "foods," is helpful, but if you really want to be motivated to avoid nonfoods, go to the back of the restaurant or store where environmentally-harmful by-products are disposed.

Reference: Meizys, Dennis, of Maryland Green Power Company, posted at mercola.com/blogs.

On Frito-Lay's website, plugs for their processed products include the statement that their foods (read "non-foods") are for fun, not for health. At least they're being somewhat honest.

Most consumers (72%) are trying to eat less trans fats. However, they are unclear about which fats are healthful. No wonder, since the news from scientists has been contradictory, confusing, and frequently changed.

Reference: "Survey Reveals Consumer 'Diet Disconnects,'" *Nutrition Week*, 4 June 2007: 37(11), 2.

Dr. Sherry A. Rogers (MD) gets as frustrated as I do about nonfoods. Why, she insists, can't the American Heart Association and Harvard Medical School and other similar organizations just come out and say what has already been proven—*that there is no safe level of trans fats?* Damaging trans fats can contribute to many maladies, from heart disease, arthritis, and allergies to cancer, MS, colitis, and "brain rot." I cringe when I see toddlers shoving animal crackers in their mouths. I seethe when I see people grabbing chips, pretzels, donuts, salad dressings, mayonnaise, pretzels, breads, cookies, and French fries off the grocery shelves. Anything that says partially-hydrogenated oil, hydrogenated oil, soy oil, soybean oil, vegetable oil, or cottonseed oil should be shunned.

Reference: Rogers, Sherry A., "American Heart Association Is a Day Late and a Pound Short," *Total Wellness*, Nov. 2006: 4.

When oil is used for frying, the temperature is raised to such a high level that a percentage of the oil is broken down and decomposes into a muck of defiled, nasty fat substances.

Did you know that you need fats in your diet in order to lose fat from your body? Not getting enough fat in your diet can contribute to your packing on the pounds. Besides, people on low-fat diets almost always consume more refined sugars. A low fat intake is also associated with high insulin resistance, a prelude to diabetes.

A Swedish study found that women who regularly consumed at least one serving of full-fat dairy products every day gained about 30% *less* weight than women who didn't.

Reference: "And Fatter?," and "Whole Fat Milk, Lower Weight Gain," *Wise Traditions*, Summer 2007: 8(2), 13.

Scientists who reviewed the scientific literature concluded that trans fats in any amount increases the risk of heart disease. In January 2006, the FDA mandated labeling of foods containing more than 500 milligrams of trans fat per serving. But you still have to read labels. Trans fats remain popular with restaurants and makers of packaged baked goods. Manufacturers and restaurants like partially hydrogenated vegetable oils (trans fats) because of their long shelf life, "buttery" taste and texture, and stability for deep-frying. I don't like them and neither should you.

Reference: *Tufts University Health & Nutrition Letter*, Aug. 2006:24(6), 6.

The average North American consumes 4.7 pounds of trans fat each year.

Reference: Food and Drug Administration and LiveScience.com.

Restaurants alone use five billion pounds of trans fat per year. Eight billion pounds are used by Americans as a whole. I hope these numbers are coming down, not going up.

Reference: DeMaria, Robert, "What You Need to Know to Avoid Partially Hydrogenated Oil," *HealthKeepers Magazine*, Summer 2007: 9(1), 35-39.

Mary Enig, PhD, who has studied fats for many years, says that saturated fats protect against the harmful effects of trans fats. Ironic, isn't it, that saturated fats may have been erroneously blamed for doing what trans fats do—contribute to cardiovascular disease?

Reference: Enig, Mary G., "Some Typical Questions and Misconceptions on Fats and Oils," *Wise Traditions*, Winter 2006: 7(4), 55-57.

Women who want to get pregnant should avoid the array of low-fat foods in the supermarket dairy case. High intake of low-fat dairy foods was linked with an increased risk of infertility in women (because of failure to ovulate). High intake of high-fat dairy foods was linked with a higher tendency to become pregnant. Sometimes I want to scream out that natural foods should be left alone the way Nature made them. Girls, your ovaries need natural fats from natural foods. And this applies whether you are 20 years old or 75 years young.

Reference: Chavarro, J.E., W.C. Willett, et al, "A Prospective Study of Dairy Foods Intake and Anovulatory Infertility," *Human Reproduction*, 28 Feb. 2007: Epub ahead of print.

Low-fat milk products have also been linked to ovarian cancer and other hormone-related disturbances.

Reference: McTaggart, Lynne, "The Low-Fat Fallacy," *What Doctors Don't Tell You*, Apr. 2007: 18(1), 3.

Oils are pressed out of seeds, nuts, grains, legumes, and olives. Heat and pressure are used to squeeze the oil out of the foods. With low heat, oils may then be filtered and sold as "unrefined" oil. High heat and high pressure, solvent extraction (dissolving the oil out of finely ground food with a toxic chemical solvent), mixing the oil with a very corrosive base to remove free fatty acids and protein-like substances (phospholipids) and minerals, degumming, bleaching, and deodorizing are all processes used to produce "refined" oils. During processing, most all the remaining minerals and vitamins are removed. The end results are oils that are bland tasting and colorless because all the goodness of the original food and oil has been obliterated. They are nutrient-deficient sources of calories and they contain weird and toxic substances.

Reference: Erasmus, Udo, *Fats that Heal, Fats that Kill*, Burnaby: Alive Books, 1993: 93-99.

If you want to become pregnant, cut out the trans fats. Women who got just 2% of their daily calories from trans fats had a 70 to 100% chance of infertility, because of lack of ovulation. So if you eat about 2,000 calories a day, this would equal about 4 grams of trans fats, or one doughnut. There is no reason to have *any* trans fats in your diet whoever you are. It is well known that trans fatty acids lead to heart disease and heart failure.

Reference: "Trans Fat Forestalls Fertility," *Vegetarian Times*, May/June 2007: 350, 16.

Researchers in Norway found that overweight men and women who were supplemented with about 3.5 grams of CLA (conjugated linoleic acid) for a year had significant decreases in body fat. CLA is a family of more than a dozen similar compounds that represent a natural, healthful trans fatty acid. Most trans fats, formed when fats are partially hydrogenated by laboratory manipulations, are bad for your health. But CLA is different because it is formed by Nature, not by human tampering. CLA has a different chemical structure that protects against cardiovascular disease, enhances the immune system, and helps prevent the accumulation of body fat.

Reference: "Study Finds CLA Helps Trim Body Fat, But Are Supplements Safe?," *Environmental Nutrition*, July 2007: 30(7), 3.

So why can some labels claim "0 grams trans fat" when the food item contains hydrogenated oils? It's because the FDA rules say that, when a product contains less than 0.5 grams (500 milligrams) of trans fat per serving, the number on the nutrition label can be rounded down to zero. But this does not make the product free of trans fat. The half-gram per serving is still there. And most North Americans usually eat more than the suggested serving size (which if often quite small). Thus, if you eat two servings, you get a gram of trans fat. Most people don't understand that four grams of trans fat a day is high, putting you at risk for all kinds of health problems from belly fat to allergies, cardiovascular disease to cancer. If you eat a doughnut for breakfast, you're getting over three grams of trans fats. A small order of French fries gets you even more, and two teaspoons of margarine provides over a gram as do two cookies that contain partially hydrogenated oil. Many people rack up more than 10 grams a day.

References: Lanzano, Lisa, "Trans Fat Trickery," *Natural Solutions*, Apr. 2008: Is.106, 33.

Rogers, Sherry A., "A Taste of Trans Fats Goes a Long Way," *Total Wellness*, March 2008: 6.

"Trans Fat Labels: How High Is High?," *Tufts University Health & Nutrition Letter*, Sept. 2008: 26(7):3.

The good news is that trans fats are being removed from many foods. Many cities, companies, and restaurants have been banning trans fatty acids. The bad news is that the substitutes for trans fatty acids, in most cases, are dubious at best. Since it is uncertain as to what to put into foods to replace trans fats, there is still industrial research going on. Prime considerations are that the replacements provide a long shelf life, don't destroy the taste of the product, and are essentially inexpensive. We won't know for years if these replacement fats or new processes for making manufactured foods will be as—or more—harmful to health as the industrial trans fats. If you don't wish to be a guinea pig, opt for unprocessed real foods and natural fats.

References: Getoff, David, "Ask the Health Professional," *Price-Pottenger Journal of Health & Healing*, Fall 2008: 32(3),20.

"Questions," *Duke Medicine HealthNews*, Nov. 2008: 14(11),12.

By the way, some natural foods such as dairy products and meats contain natural trans fatty acids. These are very different from the industrial sources of trans fatty acids and do not have the harmful health effects. The natural trans fats are formed by good bacteria in the stomachs of cows, sheep, and other ruminant animals. These natural fats may be protective to our health. Sadly, about 80% of the trans fats North Americans eat is the artificial, industrial versions.

References: "Are Natural Trans Fats as Bad for You as Man-Made Trans Fats?," *UC Berkeley Wellness Letter*, November 2008: 24(2), 7.

Chardigny, Jean-Micel, Frederic Destaillats, Corinne Malpuech-Brugere, et al, "Do Trans Fatty Acids From Industrially Produced Sources and From Natural Sources Have the Same Effect on Cardiovascular Disease Risk Factors in Health Subjects?," *American Journal of Clinical Nutrition*, March 2008: 87(3), 558-566.

Willett, Walter and Dariush Mozaffarian, "Ruminant or Industrial Sources of Trans Fatty Acids: Public Health Issue or Food Label Skirmish?," *American Journal of Clinical Nutrition*, Mar. 2008: 87(3):515-516.

If you eat less fat in your diet than you need, you could be stressing your thyroid as it tries to maintain normal blood-fat and temperature physiology. Eventually, this could lead to a pooped thyroid that secretes less thyroid hormone than you need. Your adrenal (stress) glands may secrete extra cortisol and epinephrine to help along the movement of stored fats into the blood when blood levels are too low. This could fatigue your adrenals after a while. If you eat enough fat but you are not digesting it properly, you could be in the same boat as not eating enough. Eat the amount of fat *your* body needs. Do not try to consume a fat-free diet. And if fats repeat on you or make you feel nauseous, you may not be digesting them. Get some professional help.

Reference: Cartmell, John, "Fat Nutrition and Body Temperature," *Townsend Letter*, Feb./Mar. 2007:119-120.

Wild berries—such as blueberries, cloudberries, and cowberries—are good sources of omega-3 fats, similar to wild green vegetables.

Reference: Bere, E. "Wild Berries: A Good Source of Omega-3," *European Journal of Clinical Nutrition*, 2007: 61(3), 431-433.

Because of the well known dangers of human-made trans fats, processed food makers have been scrambling to develop a replacement. One company invented a process to create "interesterified fats." Unfortunately, interesterified fats are turning out to be even worse than trans fats.

Reference: Sundram, K., T. Karupaiah, et al, "Stearic Acid-Rich Interesterified Fat and Trans-Rich Fat Raise the LDL/HDL Ratio and Plasma Glucose Relative To Palm Olein in Humans," *Nutrition and Metabolism*, 2007: 4, 3.

Nuts and seeds have been avoided for a while because they are high in fats. But evidence is piling up that they're very good for us. They even help prevent cardiovascular disease. Loaded with protein and minerals—like calcium, magnesium, potassium, copper, zinc, manganese—they may protect us from various cancers as well. Even though you may see warnings that you should not eat more than a paltry handful of nuts and seeds, because of their calories, they have been used successfully in weight loss programs. The trace element, strontium, is beginning to get the attention of scientists due to its ties with the immune system, brain activity, and intracellular functions as well as its involvement in the bonding of minerals to form strong bones. Strontium content in: grains and cereals, about 3 ppm (parts per million); vegetables, about 1.90 ppm; meats, about 2 ppm, and nuts, about *60* ppm.

Reference: Spiller, Gene, *Healthy Nuts*, Garden City Park, NY, Avery Publishing Group, 2000; and Heinerman, John, *Heinerman's Encyclopedia of Nuts, Berries, and Seeds*, West Nyack, NY: Parker Publishing Company, 1995: 59, 159, 237-238, 299-300, 302-303.

The Zuni Indians of Arizona used pumpkin seeds to get rid of certain intestinal parasites, such as tapeworm, and roundworm, among others.

Meats, Seafood, Eggs, and Milk:

Food animals are fed large amounts of grain because they grow fatter faster. Fattier beef, lamb, bison, and chicken have from one-third to three times more fat than animals raised on pasture. Meat, dairy products, and eggs from pasture-fed animals give you more omega-3 fatty acids and CLA (see previous entry) than products from grain-fed animals. Meat from animals raised on pasture gives you more vitamin E (usually 10 times more) and more carotenes (including lutein, zeaxanthin, and beta-carotene, up to hundreds of times more).

If the fat that surrounds a steak has a yellowish tint, it may indicate that the cow was grass-fed. If the fat is white, the cow was fed a corn and cereal grain diet. Grain-fed cattle have more fat, which makes for a more tender and moist steak. But it also means the animal did not exercise a lot, was not as healthy as it should have been, and its meat is not as good for you as it should be.

The majority of cows giving milk are kept in confinement dairies which offer unnatural, unhealthy environments. They are fed grains (and bovine growth hormone!) so they will produce the most amount of milk possible. Much less omega-3s, less CLA, less carotenes, less vitamin E, less B vitamins like B_6 and B_{12}, and less other nutrients are the results. Changes occur in the physical and chemical state of calcium and other minerals that affect absorption of those nutrients. The enzymes are messed up.

Certified organic milk, butter, and cheese are superior to ordinary milk products because the cows are not treated with artificial hormones or antibiotics, they are not fed pesticide-laden feeds, and they are raised in a more comfortable environment. But most organic milk is less nutritious than milk from grass-fed cows. Most organic dairies feed their cows a lot of grain, albeit organic grain. For the healthiest milk and healthiest meat, cows need more than an organic diet; they need their natural, original diet. Chickens grazing on grass, wild plants, seeds, and insects have far more nutrients in their meat and eggs. Best choices: milk products and meats from both grass-fed and organically-raised animals; chicken and eggs from organically-raised, really free-range birds.

Reference: Robinson, Jo, *Pasture Perfect: The Far-Reaching Benefits of Choosing Meat, Eggs, and Dairy Products from Grass-Fed Animals*, Vashon, WA: Vashon Island Press, 2004: 27-56.

Various studies have confirmed that the present-day feeding methods for cows using large amounts of grains have had, explains Dr. Ron Schmid, "a profound effect on the kind and abundance of bacteria found in milk, much to the detriment of the health of the animals and the quality of the milk." There are more acid-resistant, toxin-carrying bacteria in milk from heavily grain-fed, overly acidic cattle than from grass-fed animals. Raw milk or meat from grass-fed cows is so much safer than milk from animals kept in confinement and fed mostly grains and silage.

Reference: Schmid, Ron, *The Untold Story of Milk*, Washington D.C.: New Trends Publishing Inc, 2003: 303-305.

"Open and fair-minded officials need to learn," stressed Dr. Ron Schmid, "that raw milk from healthy animals, carefully produced and handled, simply does not cause disease *and* has remarkable health benefits." I agree. I have witnessed the health benefits gleaned by many people, including some who were supposedly allergic to milk, by using raw milk products.

Reference: Schmid, Ron, *The Untold Story of Milk*, Washington D.C.: New Trends Publishing Inc, 2003: 255.

Every half gallon of Grade A pasteurized milk contains more than 50 million bacteria. If you leave a cup of pasteurized milk and a cup of raw milk on your counter overnight, guess which one will contain more bacteria? The pasteurized one. The raw milk will ferment or sour—a good thing since it is then even easier to digest and provides probiotics. Pasteurized milk rots, it does not really sour.

Organic milk products have become popular, especially since the introduction of bovine growth hormone to induce increased milk production in dairy cows. Organic milk is chosen to avoid the hormone byproducts, antibiotic and other drug residues, and other toxins. However, many organic milks, creams, and other dairy items may be "ultra-pasteurized." They are submitted to high temperatures for long periods. This denatures the protein, alters the fatty acids, and diminishes or eradicates some important nutrients. Ice cream may be made with organic cream (pasteurized or ultra-pasteurized) but sweetened with plenty of refined sugars. "Organic" is infinitely better than conventional, but it's not a magic password to health. A wise consumer must look, not only to how a food is raised, but also to how the food is processed and packaged as well as the best way to prepare and store it.

Reference: Levin, Buck, *Environmental Nutrition*, Vason Island: HingePin, 1999: 278.

Homogenization is a process that breaks the fat globules in milk into very tiny particles. Fresh milk can't be homogenized until it's pasteurized because it will go rancid in a matter of minutes because the protective coating on the fat would be exposed to enzymes. Pasteurization destroys all the enzymes, so homogenization can take place without immediate rancidity. Pasteurization and homogenization change the milk sugar, denature the protein, alter the fats, and deplete the milk of nutrients like vitamin C, in addition to killing the enzymes.

Every year more vitamin C is destroyed in the pasteurization of milk than is produced by the Florida orange crop.

Reference: Simpson, Harold N., *Unhealthy Food=Unhealthy People*, Chicago: Peter Jon Simpson, 1994:57.

Velveeta is a "cheese spread" which contains about 60% water, not less than 20% butterfat, and a few gums to hold it together—plus sweeteners.

Reference: Bader, Myles H., *2001 Food Secrets Revealed*, Las Vegas, NV: Northstar Publishing, 1997: 178.

A lot of modern evidence indicates that yogurt and other fermented foods can have a wonderful influence on health and longevity. Nevertheless, the US government has long maintained the opposite, yet it is known that the biological value of milk protein increases during the culturing of yogurt. The lactic acid produced by fermentation of lactose (sugar in milk) acts as a digestive protector and a tonic to the nerves of the intestinal tract. Nutrient levels, such as those of vitamins B_2 and B_{12}, shoot up. In addition, tons of research articles are revealing the benefits of probiotics, the good bacteria in products like yogurt.

Reference: Schmid, Ron, *The Untold Story of Milk*, Washington D.C.; New Trends Publishing Inc, 2003: 324-332.]

Imitation crab meat, lobster, shrimp, and scallops are usually made from deep-ocean whitefish or pollock. These imitation shellfish contain high levels of salt and in some products MSG is used. The processing lowers the level of nutrients that would ordinarily be found in the fresh fish.

Reference: Bader, Myles H., *2001 Food Secrets Revealed*, Las Vegas, NV: Northstar Publishing, 1997: 125.

Seafood is becoming more and more of a problem because it is frequently contaminated with mercury, PCBs, dioxins, organochlorines, and other poisons and toxins from human pollution. However, we are told that eating fish is important for a healthful diet. What a choice.

Sweeteners:

Each person in the US is eating an average of almost 160 pounds of refined sugars per year. I don't eat refined sugars, so someone out there is eating more than 160 pounds a year. Soda accounts for more than a third of the refined sugar consumption. The average annual consumption of soda is about 55 gallons per person with 24% of the soda being artificially sweetened.
Reference: "Sugar Goes Pop," *UC Berkeley Wellness Letter*, Feb. 1999: 15(5), 8.

Low-carb proponents teach that sugar raises insulin levels and forces more fat into fat cells. But that's true of *only* simple, refined sugars. Sugars consumed as whole carbohydrate real foods can, in some cases, raise insulin levels *less* than beef, fish, and cheese.
Reference: *American Journal of Clinical Nutrition*, 1997: 66, 1264-1276.

Added sugars in the average North American diet come primarily from just five categories:
— Nondiet soft drinks: 28%
— Candy & sprinkle-on sugar: 17%
— Cookies, cakes, sweet baked goods: 16%
— Ice cream, frozen/sweetened yogurt: 10%
— Sweetened fruit drinks and iced tea: 8%
Reference: Pierre, Coleen, "Is Sugar Making You Fat?," *Prevention*, Jan. 2001: 118-126.

To burn off the average number of refined-sugar-related calories consumed in a month, you'd have to walk 52 miles.

A can of cola contains about 10 teaspoons of refined sugar. A bottle of sweetened iced tea may have up to 8 teaspoons.
Reference: Lynch, Sally, "Break the Sugar Habit," *Body & Soul*, Apr./May 2006: 23(3), 115-119.

How can you break the sugar habit? *First,* for a week or more, be aware of how much refined sugar you are eating and identify the places where you may not have suspected it lurches (like in breads, sauces, soups, yogurts, even ketchup). *Second,* for a few weeks, increase the amount of healthy real foods you eat and decrease the nonfoods. *Third,* go without any refined sugars for a week. When the week is over, you'll be better able to control your consumption of the stuff. You may notice some withdrawal-type symptoms during your sugar-free week, but you may also notice that you are beginning to feel better, and to feel better about yourself. You might even decide to quit consuming refined sugar. Celebrate with a fresh-fruit salad drizzled with raw honey.

High-fructose corn syrup (HFCS) is a human-made sweetener found in a wide range of processed nonfoods, from ketchup and salad dressings to cereals and crackers, as well as most all regular soda. HFCS has been around for over 30 years, during which time obesity rates have soared. The average North American downs 35 gallons of HFCS-sweetened soft drinks in a year. Since I don't drink soda, some of you out there are drinking more than 35 gallons of the stuff.
Reference: "Fight For Your Food Rights," *Eating Well*, Sept./Oct. 2007: 6(5), 16.

High-fructose corn syrup (HFCS) seems to be at least partly responsible for the rising rates of obesity and diabetes. HFCS now accounts for 40% of the caloric sweeteners added to foods and drinks. This highly refined sweetener seems to help people make pigs of themselves. For one thing, when soda manufacturers switched from sugar to HFCS (which is sweeter), they used the same quantity, so sodas today are a lot sweeter than they were 30 years ago. The intense sweetness can make you crave other sweet foods. Second, your body processes HFCS different from other refined sugar. For example, it doesn't produce a normal rise in insulin, which prevents the usual increase in levels of a hormone called leptin. Leptin makes you feel full so you stop eating. Too little leptin and you eat too much. If you see "high-fructose corn syrup" on a label, put the item back on the shelf.
References: Bray, G.A., S.J. Nielsen, et al, "Consumption of High-Fructose Corn Syrup in Beverages May Play a Role in the Epidemic of Obesity," *The American Journal of Clinical Nutrition*, Apr. 2004: 79(4), 537-543.
Krilanovich, Nicholas J., "Fructose Misuse, the Obesity Epidemic, the Special Problems of the Child, and a Call To Action," *American Journal of Clinical Nutrition*, Nov. 2004: 80(5), 1446-1447.]
Tallmadge, Katherine, "Is Sugar Really That Bad?", *Vegetarian Times*, Nov./Dec. 2004: 326, 30-34.
www.rense.com, 17 Dec. 2005, citing *Nature Clinical Practice Nephrology*, Dec. 2005, and online edition of the *American Journal of Physiology-Renal Physiology*.

"Evaporated cane juice" is simply dried whole juice from the sugar cane. It doesn't have the disruptive effects in the body as does refined sugar. But "organic milled sugar" or "organic sugar" is *refined* sugar. It is devoid of its balancing and synergistic nutrients that assist the body to properly handle the sugar component. "Organic evaporated cane juice" is whole. Refined sugars are just sucrose, carbohydrates missing all their essential co-workers.

Are artificial sweeteners better than refined sugars? I don't like *artificial anything* when it comes to what I put in my body. These sweeteners certainly don't appear to have helped the ever-expanding American waistline. They fool the body into thinking sugars are coming, disrupting normal biochemistry. Even though there is still a lot of controversy surrounding artificial sweeteners, some more than others, I can't believe they can be anything but upsetting to our bodies and our health.

Aspartame (aka NutraSweet, Equal, and Spoonful) accounts for 75% of adverse reactions to food additives reported to the FDA. Although a firestorm of claims made on the Internet about horrible consequences of consuming aspartame have not been supported by studies, I'd weigh on the cautious and avoid it. Many people I know felt so much better after quitting the stuff. One woman, an artist, claimed she lost her eyesight because of drinking several sodas a day sweetened with Equal. Nothing else could account for the damage to her ocular nerves. Dr. H.J. Roberts has done a formidable amount of research on aspartame. One thing he found through his own patients who had hypoglycemia (low blood sugar) is that, when they stopped using it, most of them made remarkable recoveries.

> Reference: Howard, Brian C., "Sugar or Sweetener?, *E Magazine*, Mar./Apr. 2006: 17(2), 40-41, and Roberts, H.J., *Aspartame Disease*, West Palm Beach, FL. Sunshine Sentinel Press, 2001.

Splenda (sucralose) claims it is "made from sugar so it tastes like sugar." This is misleading—it is not a "natural" sugar. It may start out as sugar, but then laboratory manipulations replace one group of atoms with another. Specifically, chlorine atoms are forced onto it, making it a chlorinated hydrocarbon. I wouldn't want that in my body, and I don't think you do either. The body doesn't recognize it as a sugar or a carbohydrate. It can't be metabolized by the body, so it's considered calorie-free. But, do we want to put chemicals into our body that that are alien to it? This is a synthetic chemical cooked up in a flask in a laboratory somewhere. Animal research has shown that it can cause shrinkage of the thymus gland, enlargement of the liver and kidneys, wasting of lymph follicles, decreased red blood cell count, diarrhea, and other ills.

> Reference: "Is Splenda Sugar-Coating the Facts?," *Tufts University Health & Nutrition Letter*, July 2005: 23(5), 8, and Hull, Janet Starr, *www.splendaexposed.com*

Got a sweet tooth? A study found that fruit may satisfy your cravings instead of refined sugars. People who eat lots of sweets like candy and cookies tend to prefer fruit more than people who want salty snacks.

> Reference: "Candy Lovers Also Favor Fruit," *Tufts University Health & Nutrition Letter*, Oct. 2006: 24(6), 3.

A non-diet soft drink is loaded with refined sugars. You knew that. But did you know that breaking down the sugar in your body requires water? This means that you will probably be thirstier than before you grabbed that soft drink. Alcoholic drinks require a cup of water per drink to metabolize the alcohol. If you're thirsty, the best thing to drink is good, clean water.

> Reference: Bader, Myles H., *2001 Food Secrets Revealed*, Las Vegas, NV: Northstar Publishing, 1997: 194.

Chewing gums nowadays are made from synthetic polymers, mostly styrene-butadiene rubbers and polyvinyl acetate. The end product is composed of 60% sugar, 20% corn syrup, and 20% actual gum material.

> Reference: Bader, Myles H., *2001 Food Secrets Revealed*, Las Vegas, NV: Northstar Publishing, 1997: 134.

Honey is a health food. It sustains energy for athletes and helps muscles recuperate faster post-workout. It may help prevent heart disease by slowing the oxidation (breakdown) of LDL cholesterol. And applying it to the skin can speed the healing of wounds. It may slow the growth of dental plaque too. Eating honey can raise your blood levels of polyphenols, which are linked to decreased risks of heart disease, cancer, and stroke. Get really *raw* honey, not the cooked, refined versions.

Reference: O'Connor, Amy, "Oh, Honey!", *Organic Style*, May 2005: 5(4), 92-96; and *Health*, Sept. 2004: 18(7), 66.

Until the end of the Middle Ages, honey was the favored sweetener in much of the world, yet not the only one. Date sugar (dried pulverized dates) or syrup, fig syrup, malted grains (sprouted, dried or roasted, and finely ground, such as barley malt), grape juice, and whole sugar cane juice were among sweeteners used in various countries. These are still good sweeteners as long as they are not refined, overcooked, or otherwise messed with. Native Americans made maple syrup for hundreds of years before the coming of Europeans. The sap is boiled for a long time to make syrup which retains its mineral content.

Reference: Onstad, Diane, *Whole Foods Companion*, White River Junction, VT: Chelsea Green Publishing Company, 1996: 453, 463.

Although dieticians and others are fond of saying that honey and these other sweeteners are "just sugar"—no different from the refined sugars so prevalent in our modern nonfoods—they miss an important point. We are not saying that real natural sweeteners are packed with lots of nutrients, even though they do contain small amounts of a variety of them. But they do contain enough nutrients and other food factors that help your body to properly use the sugars without seriously disrupting the biochemistry. Over the years, for example, I have seen diabetics who were able to use small amounts of really raw honey, particularly Tupelo, without disturbing their blood sugar or insulin. I can't say every diabetic can do this since each individual is unique. I can say that, in my experience, real natural sweeteners do not appear to cause the same problems as refined or artificial versions.

Once fructose is separated from whole fruits or other foods, it's just another refined sugar. Actually, it's just another ultra-refined sugar. It can mess with your blood sugar metabolism, among other things. The same applies to xylitol and D-mannose which are also refined carbohydrates. Both seem to have some health benefits, but what happens with long-term use of large amounts of these two simple sugars are not yet known. "Brown sugar" is nothing more than refined white sugar with a bit of molasses added to it. "Raw sugar" is not raw—it's coarse refined white sugar. "Turbinado sugar" is coarse white sugar named after the turbine in which it is refined. Refined sugars have never had good track records when it comes to human health.

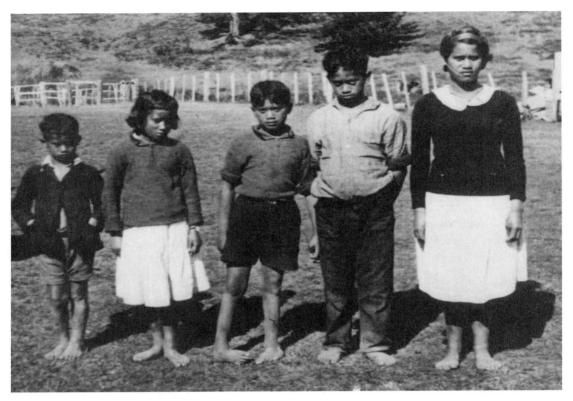

These photographs were taken by Dr Weston A Price. They illustrate a few of the many physical differences that occur from food consumed during pregnancy and early childhood. The photo shows five children in a New Zealand Maori family.

The oldest girl (on the right) has a typical Maori pattern of face whereas the two younger brothers next to her have progressive distortions in their facial features. The girl has normally-formed feet, the middle boy has flat feet, and the third child has clubbed feet. The mother ate a traditional, whole real food diet when pregnant with the girl. The girl was raised on a natural diet and was not exposed to what Dr Price called "foods of commerce"—refined, processed nonfoods. The girl's brother next to her was conceived while the mother was eating a native, natural diet, but as an infant he was exposed to nonfoods. The center child was conceived and born on "foods of commerce." Obviously, things got progressively worse. Now look at the final two Maori children. The girl was conceived on "foods of commerce," but born and raised on a natural diet. The last little boy was conceived and born totally on a natural, native diet and was never exposed to nonfoods.

Notice the narrowing of the face due to the narrower dental arch especially in the middle child. The shape of the head in the two boys raised on a diet of highly refined, over-processed nonfoods has a distinct look. The children born and raised on a natural, whole foods diet are more robust, healthy-looking.

88

Here are four photographs taken by Dr Weston Price of Polynesians who were isolated from the influence of modern industrialized foods. They are a happy, beautiful people, physically strong, and have splendid physiques. Being a dentist, Dr Price was particularly interested in the mouth and teeth. The people shown here ate their natural, native diet, depending much on the sea for food. They have healthy features and essentially perfect teeth.

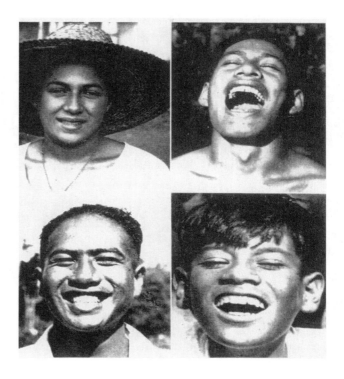

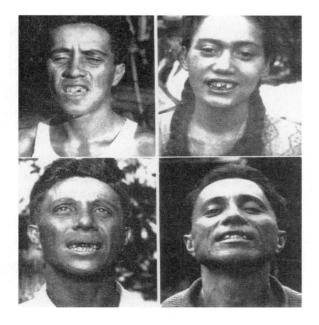

In this photograph we see four more Polynesians, typical of the "modernized" islanders. They represent the Polynesians who ceased to depend on their native foods which had been displaced by imported refined nonfoods. Dr Price observed ships at the islands exchanging white refined flour and refined sugar for the natives' copra (coconut meat from which coconut oil could be extracted). Tooth decay ran rampant where as the natives eating their natural diet had virtually none. These peoples who converted to nonfoods became sick in many ways, just as we commonly see in our own country.

89

Chapter Six

WHICH DIET DO I FOLLOW?

Low-carb, high-fat, high-protein? Low-fat, high-carb? Mediterranean? Macrobiotic? My "type" determined by Aureveda or blood or metabolism or some other way? Caveman? Vegetarian? Vegan? Raw food? Movie-star endorsed? Diet guru-based? Clinically-based?

And the answer is: I don't know.

However, there are a couple of things I *do* know: (1) Each and every one of us needs *all* nutrients—all the vitamins, minerals, amino acids, fatty acids, and every other food nutrient, both known and unknown. (2) We need to eat wholesome, real foods that are as close as possible to how Nature made them and avoid industrialized nonfoods and unfoods as much as possible. (See chapter: "What's in Your Mouth?") (3) To get the answers about your unique personal needs, you should pay attention to your own body. You may need help in learning how to do this and how to interpret your body's messages, but your very own body knows more than anyone else what is best for you.

Notice I said to pay attention to your own *body*, not your mind. Your mind can be influenced by all the media reports, expert advice or scientific studies which, in themselves, can be contradictory or confusing. For example, for years we have been told to avoid fats in our diet, but that turned out to be a big mistake. Not only have people become more deficient in nutrients they need from fats, but many have gained weight, developed blood sugar problems like diabetes, and gotten into other negative health issues as a result. Yet some folks still unnecessarily harbor a fear of fat. Or, our minds may perpetuate habits such as the way we ate as we grew up or the habits we accumulated over the years. Or our minds may use foods to create numbness, for rewards or comfort, to avoid loneliness, depression or anxiety. Our minds may rationalize or justify what we eat or when we eat, like skipping lunch so we can gorge at night in front of the television.

Your body doesn't care about all this. It knows what it needs and, if we learn to listen—if we can just get back in touch with our bodies—it will give us the clues.

You see, you are singular, unique, individual. Outside of eating wholesome, real foods, what your very own distinctive body needs is special and different from that of other people. There is no "average" person. World-renowned biochemist Roger Williams, PhD, called it "biochemical individuality." How we relate to our environment, how we relate to drugs or chemicals, alcohol or sugar, fats or proteins or carbohydrates, reflects our anatomical, physiological, biochemical, and genetic individuality. Each of us does need every nutrient, but the amounts and natural forms that each of us needs differ. Dr. Williams found differences of anywhere from 30% to 500% in (blood or saliva) nutritional values and in nutrient needs of individuals. Some doctors have even estimated that nutritional requirements can vary from person to person a thousand-fold or more. To be optimally healthy, one person will need more of one particular nutrient than another person, and less of some other nutrient than someone else. You may become deficient in certain nutrients because you don't get enough of them in your diet, or your unique biochemistry may simply require additional amounts of some nutrients for the biochemical pathways to function properly.

What is the optimal diet? Joseph Pizzorno, ND, answers with "it depends." It depends on your genetic heritage, your personal health history, your environmental stresses, your lifestyle, what you have eaten all your life, your unique needs, and "myriad other factors." The mixing of ethnicities means we're no longer "optimized" for a specific type of diet.

Dr. Pizzorno and many more of us who connect with real people are sure of only two things: (1) Eating refined, processed, nutritionally-deficient, distorted nonfoods, often containing foreign chemicals, will contribute to disease and ill health. This is food forgery, food fiction. (2) Eating honest-to-goodness real food, made by cooperating with Nature, processed as little as possible, chuck-full of nutrients and other food factors, will promote wellness and health vitality. This is food fidelity, food fact. Do you know that the foods most commonly consumed in this country are beef (from unnaturally fed cattle), processed meats (like deli meats or hotdogs), refined-grain bakery products, eggs (from unnaturally raised chickens), French fries, pasteurized dairy products, and sweets and other desserts? This nonfood preponderance does not add up to health, even if you think these things taste good. Although humans are adaptable, we cannot adapt *healthfully* to nonfood. Whatever we eat—and this is highly individualized—should be whole, natural, and fresh.

The way you eat, what you eat, even when you eat are best determined according to what your body tries to tell you. Not only what your taste tells you, but how you feel from eating certain foods will help you know your needs. Over the years, I have known individuals who felt best eating lots of organic meats, seafood, and dairy products with some vegetables and fruits thrown in. I have worked with individuals who discovered their energy and vitality improved when they switched to a vegetarian diet. On the other hand, some individuals discovered just the opposite—that a vegetarian diet made them feel worse. Eating lots of fatty foods makes some people lethargic, while others feel stronger and peppier. I have known individuals who said that their bodies want vegetables more than fruits, fruits more than vegetables, red meats more than poultry or seafood, poultry or seafood more than red meats, grains more than meats, meats more than grains. You get the picture.

Your very own physiology and biochemistry will respond to foods, and even nonfoods, differently. Refined sugars will wreak havoc on the blood sugar metabolism of most all people, yet some react more than others, perhaps becoming diabetic. Refined flours and sugars will make the blood triglycerides spike higher on some folks than others. A couple of cups of coffee a day can be handled by most people, maybe giving them a bit of a buzz, but some people aren't affected by five or six or more cups. Others can't deal with a single cup without suffering from sleeplessness, anxiety, or even panic attacks. I recall one man who would drink a cup of coffee and then fall asleep.

Many "prescribed" diets can be too restrictive or even unhealthy for some folks. For example, the raw food diet has been invigorating and health-enhancing for some people, yet it can be extremely limiting and lead to deficiencies and difficulties for others. (I should interject something here: including some raw foods into our diets is important for everyone. *How much* varies according to the individual, but definitely a good amount. Cooking destroys or denatures some nutrients. Temperatures above 114 degrees Fahrenheit also destroy the enzymes that help you process or metabolize food components, absorb nutrients, and obtain the most energy from the food. But, obviously, not all foods can be eaten raw). Trying to eat a vegan diet can lead to B_{12}, zinc, and other nutritional deficits in some people, but not others. A high-fat, high-protein, low-carbohydrate diet has made some individuals nauseous and sick, deficient in many vitamins and minerals, whereas others may thrive on it.

There are those of you who feel well eating "three square" meals a day, whereas there are others of you who are better at being "grazers," eating five, six, or more small meals a day. Some of you can't bear the thought of eating first thing in the morning—you may want some nourishment by mid-morning—but some of you wake up hungry. Some people who skip breakfast because they are "too busy" to eat, feel for the rest of the day like a truck ran over them and gouge themselves later in the day.

Craving some food or foods indicates something. If you desire chocolate or salty foods, for instance, it may mean your adrenal glands are stressed or fatigued. If you long for fats, you may be deficient in some fat-soluble vitamins or essential fatty acids, or you may not be digesting fats properly (I remember one client who would sit down with a spoon and devour a jar of mayonnaise). If you are a woman and you start to drool just thinking about a nice juicy steak, perhaps you are iron-deficient, or maybe you haven't been getting enough protein. Some of us may not be able to get enough green leafy vegetables because we can best absorb the minerals and vitamins from these foods, or we need more of certain phytochemicals than do other people. I recall one lady who couldn't satisfy her desire for onions because she needed lots of sulfur. You could crave certain foods because they contain nutrients you need, or the craving may be an indication of something imbalanced or skewed going on in your body. There may be times when a food you usually eat becomes repugnant to you for a while. Listen!

Your body will indicate if changes in the seasons, changes in circumstances, changes in health matters, life transitions, stress levels, or any other changes mean you should change what and how you eat. Most of us want more fruits and vegetables, like big salads, during warmer seasons, and rib-sticking grains, soups, beans, or meats during cold months. Listen to your body because what you need will change from time to time. Take an extreme example: Perhaps one of the ultimate health issues we fear is cancer, a huge change in our lives. There are cancer patients who have made a complete recovery on a Macrobiotic diet (a vegetarian, mostly-cooked diet), whereas others have done better on many raw foods (including lots of freshly-made juices). Some cancer victims who have progressed well on a vegetarian-type diet will suddenly begin to desire meats and other animal foods. Following this clue, they continue to do well. If folks with cancer experience changed needs along their paths, then surely those of us with less horrific problems will also experience changed needs.

Even when it comes to weight loss, no trendy plan or program can claim better results than another. When the results are weighed in, there are no significant differences in pounds shed. There are differences, however, in how people feel and how their individual biochemistries respond while on the diet and in the future.

We may need the support and guidance of a nutritionist, doctor, or other knowledgeable health professional. But, this should be as a companion or attendant on our journey in discovering what our own bodies are trying to tell us, in "reading" the clues (if we can't figure them out for ourselves). Too many people completely turn their health decisions, including their diets, over to someone else—a physician, for example—when, in reality, our own health is not only our own responsibility, but it is also something that our own bodies know better how to attain. A wise health professional will help us determine what our bodies are trying to communicate rather than simply imposing a certain diet, set of rules or treatments on us.

Keep in mind that for every food there is on the face of this earth, there is some nutritionist or doctor or scientist who believes it is toxic and should never be eaten. I have read books written by or personally spoken to hundreds of "experts," each with his/her own opinion of what should or should not be consumed as healthful food. Every single one is right, and every single one is wrong. What each one claims *is* correct for him/herself, and perhaps some other people, definitely is *not* correct for everyone. They point to history, but historical evidence is replete with different diets that sustained different peoples. No one truly knows exactly what our ancestors ate because variety, location, circumstances, and needs were determining factors. Besides, most everyone is now a 'blend' of many ethnicities.

Annemarie Colbin warned about the "fallacy of being stuck in *any* single, strict food ideology." Even people who have made conscientious dietary changes to "health food" can become stuck in doctrine and cease listening to the signals from their own bodies. There is no one diet that is correct for everyone all the time.

Health professionals who recommend diets and/or supplements must keep this in mind as well. Joseph Pizzorno, ND, brought up the question of *how* natural products should be prescribed. "The answer," he says, is "not for the disease, but for the person." There is a need to understand where a person's unique physiology and unique biochemistry is imbalanced or dysfunctional, why this is so, which nutritional therapies will be most effec-tive for that individual, and what bumps may occur along the road so that the person can best be helped. We need to avoid any tendency toward "cookbook" nutrition—"recipes" of diet or supplements that we think will work the same way for every individual. Your needs are different from mine. We each—perhaps with some insight and assistance from a knowledgeable health professional—must find our own nutritional nook. In this area, each of us can say, like the song, "I did it *my* way."

Congratulations! You are now free of diet dogma. You can personalize a relationship to food and nutrition. It may seem a bit scary at first but with freedom comes responsibil-ity. Remember, you can get some guidance from a knowledgeable health professional. But, go ahead and take the first step—introduce yourself to your own body, begin to communicate, and develop a lovely friendship. You will never have a better or closer friend.

References

Colbin, Annemarie, *Food and Healing*, New York: Ballantine Books, 1986/1996.

DeCava, Judith A., "Food Fights, Part I," and "Food Fights, Part II," *Nutrition News and Views*, May/June 2001: Vol.5, No.3:1-8 and Jul./Aug. 2001: Vol.5, No.4:1-8.

"Evaluating 4 Diets from A(tkins) to Z(one) *Environmental Nutrition,* June 2007: Vol.30, No.6:3.

Nestle, Marion, *What to Eat*, New York: North Point Press, 2006.

Onstad, Dianne, *Whole Foods Companion*, White River Junction, VT: Chelsea Green Publishing Company, 1996.

Pizzorono, Joseph, "What IS the Optimal Diet?," *Integrative Medicine*, Aug./Sept. 2006: Vol.5, No.4:6-7.

Pizzorno, Joseph, "Why Faddism Fails," *Integrative Medicine*, June/July 2007:Vol.6, No.3:8-9.

Santillo, Humbart, *Intuitive Eating*, Prescott, AZ: Hohm Press), 1993.

Williams, Roger J., *Biochemical Individuality*, New Canaan, CT: Keats Publishing, 1956/1998.

Wright, Jonathan V., "Food for Thought," *Nutrition & Healing*, Mar. 2006: Vol.13, Is.2:5.

FOOD FOR THOUGHT

The desire for change shows up in your body, not just in your thoughts. Pay attention to what it is trying to tell you.

Each of us has more than 80,000 enzyme systems in our bodies and each performs a specialized function. Enzymes are much more than catalysts. They're the "labor force" that builds your body—similar to the construction workers who build your house. They contain a life energy not found in mere catalysts. The activity factor of enzymes has never been synthesized in any laboratory.

Reference: Howell, Edward, *Food Enzymes for Health & Longevity*, Twin Lakes WI: Lotus Press, 1994: 12, 17.

There is a difference between cooked calories and raw calories. Dr. Edward Howell observed, in his work, that "it was impossible to get people fat on raw foods, regardless of the calorie intake."

Reference: Howell, Edward, *Food Enzymes for Health & Longevity*, Twin Lakes WI: Lotus Press, 1994:21.

While we all need some raw foods, eating an exclusively raw-food diet can be too restrictive. Its followers "are at risk for deficiencies of vitamin B_{12} and omega-3 fatty acids if they don't take supplements," says Andrea N. Giancoli, MPH, RD. Cooking definitely destroys some nutrients, but it may make others more absorbable such as the lycopene in tomatoes and the beta-carotene in carrots.

Reference: Stamos, Jenny, "The Raw-food Diet," *Eating Well*, Oct./Nov. 2006: Vol.5, No.5:19

The idea that the four major blood types evolved in different environments and therefore predispose people to different nutritional needs was popularized by Peter D'Adamo in his 1996 book, *Eat Right 4 Your Type*. But blood type actually has little to do with body chemistry or digestion. Since the A, AB, B, and O blood-type groups were identified early in the 1920s, some 200 different blood group substances have been identified and grouped within 19 different systems. The genes for blood type are not related to the genes that handle the food we eat. Yes, our ethnic background may have an influence on what we need in foods. But, these days, no one is a pure-bred anything. We must listen to our own special needs.

Reference: "Is There Any Relationship Between Blood Type and Nutrition?," *Tufts University Health & Nutrition Letter,* Oct. 2006: Vol.24, No.6:7.

A study that followed almost 50,000 women over eight years found that a diet low in fat but high in fruit, vegetables, and grains—the type of diet we've been told will protect us from disease—doesn't significantly reduce the risk of breast cancer, colorectal cancer, or cardiovascular disease in postmenopausal women. These women, being older, were at high risk for all these diseases, but following a low-fat diet didn't really help.

Reference: "Study Examines Low-fat Diet, Ailments in Women," *Nutrition Week,* 13 Feb. 2006: Vol.36, No.4:2.

Low-fat diets are not created equal. It's not just the amount of fat; it's the type of fat you eat that's important. Eating trans fats, refined oils, fake fats, rancid fats, and fats heated at very high temperatures (as in deep frying) does damage to your body. Natural, unaltered, fresh real fats not only won't cause damage, they are important assets to your health.

Cravings aren't only possible signals of a lack of a certain nutrient or a glitch in our systems. Eating urges can also be linked to cues in the environment. The time of day: is it near mealtime or does watching a particular TV show make you think it's time for a snack? Where you are: walking past a food court or running into the grocery store to "just" get some paper towels can bring on the munchies. Emotional memories, fatigue, boredom, being mentally exhausted, depression, loneliness—any or all can trigger a desire to eat. Different people crave different things at different times for different reasons.

Reference: Hobbs, Suzanne Havala, "How Can I Conquer Food Cravings?," *Vegetarian Times,* Feb. 2007: Is.347:31-32.

In its annual snacking poll, *Fitness* magazine reports that 39% of us tear into a bag of chips and 25% dip into cookies or candy. Only 19% bite into healthy snacks such as fruit, nuts, or yogurt. At work, people stash snacks into their desk drawers: 1. candy/gum, 2. chips, 3. chocolate.

Reference: O'Brien, Pamela, "2nd Annual Snacking Poll," *Fitness,* Apr. 2007: 69.

Real food has the power to transform and to heal. Which foods will you choose?

Chapter Seven

SUPPLEMENTS:
IS THERE A DIFFERENCE?

Many of us are old enough to remember the slogan, "Better Living through Chemistry." As far as our health was concerned, it expressed the notion that scientists could devise or formulate anything needed for our concerns regarding well-being and treat any diseases from acne to aging, colds to cancer. Science, it was thought, was one-up on Nature. However, the truth is that your body is smarter than scientists.

For years, scientists told us that the human body doesn't know the difference between separated or chemical-imitation nutrients and natural, whole-food nutrients. Well, numerous scientific studies (and decades of seeing the effects on countless people, which, as we all know, doesn't count in the "scientific method" rules) are proving this concept is wrong. Your body *does* know the difference.

Most scientists work by what is called reductionism. They assume that, by breaking down something from Nature into smaller and smaller parts—cutting it up into little pieces—they can study these parts in detail. This analysis of parts and their interactions with each other have led to most technological advances we now enjoy. We could call this the main strength of science. However, there are serious weaknesses in these assumptions that have become more apparent in recent years, especially when they are applied to living humans and real foods. One big one is that scientists can't put the parts back together and they haven't grasped the intricate interweaving of the whole. There is a quality that exists with the entire organization, the harmony, the synchronicity of the whole.

Another weakness that is becoming evident in separating or imitating nutrient parts is that some compounds in foods, plants, and animals may be present in miniscule amounts—

parts per million or even parts per billion or trillion—yet they still exert a huge amount of "bioactivity." In other words, teeny, tiny amounts of substances being discovered play an important part in how a food affects living tissues within itself and, when we eat it, within us. If those minute ingredients are missing, the food doesn't work the same. There's even more. When these teeny, tiny amounts of substances are combined with teeny, tiny amounts of other substances that naturally occur in a real food, the effect, the power, the energy is increased substantially, sometimes by several orders of magnitude. For example, phytochemicals—plant substances, many of which are just now being identified—can occur in various numbers, combinations, and amounts. They all work together and work with each and every other substance in the plant. There is a synergy which makes the whole a much greater entity than the sum of all its parts. There are thousands of phytochemicals, many still unknown. For instance, more than 300 carotenoids and more than 4000 flavonoids are presently known to exist in food. There are many thousands of other substances in foods, some still unknown. A leaf of spinach, for example, contains more than 10,000 different components. Other foods may be even more complex, containing even more interwoven parts.

Now, think about taking out one of these parts, or worse still, making a synthetic imitation. Will it work the same as the whole package of natural substances? Of course not, yet we have been told these imitation nutrient parts will work the same as whole natural ones. Once a compound in a food is removed from its living context, broken off from the natural matrix within which it exists, it is no longer what many scientists believe it is. Such unnatural separations can never produce the outcome they want—the nourishment needed for wellbeing.

Everything the scientists decide or conclude based on that separation and fragmentation will always end up wrong. Your body knows this and now an ever-increasing number of scientific studies indicate that the separation or synthetic imitation of a part will not work like those in real food complexes. They are an inadequate and incomplete method of supplying nutrients which certainly do not match Nature's intricate complexities and harmony. Foods are complete packages of interwoven ingredients.

Since there are so many components to foods and many of them are still unknown, why would we want to add separated nutrient bits and pieces into our diet, one or a few at a time, rather than getting the benefits of the whole foods? We would be cheating ourselves of many food factors. And, as nutrients and other food components interact synergistically or symbiotically, we'd miss out on all that needed interaction.

Nutrients are embedded in a complex web of precisely balanced interconnections. Nutrients, food, our bodies and health, are *all* intricate systems of interconnections. Some scientists, like professors David R. Jacobs, PhD, and Linda C. Tapsell, PhD, are now arguing for the need to study and focus on whole foods rather than individual, separated nutrients. They understand that the history of looking at and using separated nutrients "tends to oversimplify a complex system and has even done harm." Identifying specific

100

SUPPLEMENTS: IS THERE A DIFFERENCE?

"bioactive components" in food may be helpful, but such information is incomplete.

An academic review, conducted by the University of Minnesota School of Public Health, concluded that food as a whole is the key to a healthy diet. Professor David Jacobs, PhD, the principal investigator, said, "We are confusing ourselves and the public by talking so much about nutrients when we should be talking about foods." Professor Jacobs and other researchers are now calling attention to the fact that the single-nutrient approach to nutrition has not been shown to improve people's health, and that even long-term randomized clinical trials—considered best for determining the best nutrition—have also failed to prove that nutrition parts are beneficial. We (and nutrition scientists) need to think in terms of whole foods in whole diets. Supplements, if needed, should also consist of whole foods because whole foods are far more beneficial to health than are separated parts, and light years more beneficial than synthetic parts.

Michael Pollan, in his book, *In Defense of Food*, refers to the reductionistic, parts-is-parts approach to nutrition that has been used by scientists for decades as "nutritionism" (a term coined by an Australian sociologist of science). Don't confuse "nutritionism" with "nutrition." The "ism" means it's not a scientific subject, but an ideology, a system of ideas or assumptions. This ideology has tried to convince us that the most important thing is not the food but the "nutrient," and that because you and I can't see the nutrients, we need scientists to tell us what to eat. Thus, we must attempt to eat "scientifically" in order to fulfill a myopic view or notion of health. If we don't eat "right," then we can take supplements made of nutrient parts to make up for what we are missing. In a nutshell, we have been led to believe that foods are basically the sum of their nutrient parts. This is wrong because there is so much more to the story. For one thing, the interaction of all the parts—nutrients or not, know or unknown—is absolutely essential.

All the naturally-occurring ingredients in whole foods and their interactions make up a *matrix* which influences all the biological processes that need to take place in our bodies to ensure our health. This interaction represents synergy in which all the players are needed to participate in a harmonious concert.

When we bring up the subject of food synergy, it's important to understand the difference between a food and a drug. All real foods come from living things, plants or animals. Living things are extremely complex. The vast majority of components of plants and animals are functional, having some kind of purpose, exerting some sort of meaningful activity, and are kept in balance. Thus, thousands of substances in a food matrix must be considered as probably having biological activity that benefits our health as consumers of the food. All these substances work with each other and balance each other, so it would be extremely simplistic to evaluate the effect of or consume only single food ingredients. We need the whole package.

On the other hand, drugs are isolated substances, even if they are taken from foods or herbs. Professors Jacobs and Tapsell write: "Many supplements derived from food are

101

isolated substances, such as *B*-carotene (beta-carotene) and could therefore be classified as drugs." Even placing a separated or manufactured "nutrient" in foods ("enriching" or "fortifying")—like adding *B*-sitostanol to margarine, calcium to orange juice, folic acid to bakery products—means that these substances were not and are not part of the food matrix and don't have the same biologic action as if they were naturally an integrated part of the food. Putting it bluntly, taking individual, separated, or imitation "nutrients" is tantamount to taking drugs whether they are added to foods or taken in pills or powders. They are *not* integrated—naturally combined, unified, in symmetry—with the rest of the naturally-occurring compounds in real foods and they don't act the same in your body as a real food matrix.

Also, when you take a "high potency" vitamin, mineral, amino acid, or whatever, (we're talking about the isolated, fabricated, or nonfood supplements that dominate the market) you're not getting what you may think. You probably assume that "high potency" means more effectiveness, more power, increased capability. Actually, real whole food complexes—the packages that Nature provides, not the singled-out chemicals that humans separate or artificially imitate—exert far more healthful influence on your body's cells. The "high potency" individual chemicals only provide a higher drug effect, not a food effect. The higher the drug effect, the more your body has to deal with these foreign substances, and this can mean even toxic effects and harm.

When one part of a food is extracted or imitated, it's no longer natural. It may be called a nutrient, but it can't be used in our bodies in the same way that a whole nutritional package can. No plant or animal in Nature consists of just one part. Ingesting a part by itself in large amounts does not produce the same results as consuming a whole food in which that particular nutrient occurs. Saying one part of a food is the most important part is like saying the roof is the most important part of a house and we don't have to pay much attention to the rest of the structure. Without the other house parts, like the foundation and walls, and without those parts being in the correct positions to serve their proper purposes, the house is not serviceable. The roof tumbles down. The whole thing is just a pile of materials. It doesn't work. The same applies to using isolated, and especially synthetic or manufactured, nutrients. In fact, I can't think of them as real nutrients.

Science has learned so much and has helped to make incredible advances in many areas yet, the scientific method is limited. One professor put it this way: "You can ask us anything about death; we scientists are specialists when it comes to death and matter. But if you want to know something about life, you're barking up the wrong tree." Taking a living thing apart and scrutinizing its many components does not give you a picture of *life*—how all the thousands, millions, or even billions of participatory parts all act together, how they are all infused with a life force, how they all together fit into a complex environment with other living and inert things. The scientific method disrupts and destroys the *ecology* of plants, soil, water, animals, and humans: the intricate symbiotic interrelationships wherein disturbing one part affects all the other parts and the whole.

When nutrient parts or manufactured imitations are used, numerous problems exist. Here are some of them:

1. A part or imitation may be a *different* chemical from the natural, food form.
2. A part or imitation may have a different "optical structure" from the natural form. It can be a *mirror image* in its chemical structure, like trying to put a right-handed glove on your left hand.
3. It may have the same formula as far as molecules go, but it will be *different* in its physical and chemical properties. It won't function in the same way. For example, some vitamins (like many of the B vitamins on the market) are made from coal tar. Yes, tar obtained by distilling coal which is commonly used for dyes, drugs, and other industrial items that have absolutely no relationship to foods. The coal tar can be constructed into a formula that duplicates one nutrient part, like a B vitamin, but it is a far cry from the real food complex. Maybe cockroaches, supposedly able to eat anything, could live on coal tar chemicals, but humans can't.
4. It will be *only one* member of a large group of variously-structured compounds that all need to work together for optimal nutritional effects.
5. Using the process of *synthesis*—forming copies of separated nutrients in a laboratory—means not only is the nutrient a fake imitation, but there is also the possibility of contamination from other chemicals.
6. Taking large amounts of one isolated nutrient separated from a group or complex often inhibits absorption of other group members or other nutrients. Synthetic (manufactured from non-food sources) and isolated (chemically extracted from a food or other source) vitamins *are not absorbed, assimilated, and used as effectively* as nutrients in their natural, complex state (real food). Minerals extracted from rocks, soil, coral, or other non-food sources are also not used in the body as well as minerals from foods.
7. Large amounts of a single, separated nutrient can increase or *mask* the need for other nutrients.
8. Taking large amounts of a nutrient part or imitation can *displace* other nutrients that normally accompany it in real foods. In other words, you end up creating deficiencies of members of the nutrient group that have been left out. For example, taking large amounts of ascorbic acid (often called "vitamin C") can create deficits of copper, rutin, and/or flavonoids—natural associates of ascorbic acid in real foods.
9. A nutrient is normally and naturally a group of substances, a complex, network, ensemble—a package of ingredients all working together. It is *never isolated* in Nature. It is never a single thing. "Pure" vitamin C—aka ascorbic acid—is fabricated from refined corn syrup or sugar, not from whole food. It's about as far away from being a food as you can get. It is isolated, devoid of the active, synergistic co-workers inherent in real foods. It can't support life because it is a chemical with no food value.
10. Nutrients require *other* nutrients to be activated, balanced, operative, and nourishing. The "chemically-pure" vitamin (a part), for example, has its biological activity (function) destroyed. The "elemental" mineral—one from a non-food

source like calcium from rock—cannot be used in the body like one that has been prepared by plants for use as food. Minerals from broccoli or cheese have been prepared by the broccoli plant or cow so we can use them as nutrients, as food. Eating rocks or pieces of coral to get calcium will hardly have the same effect. They are not human foods. In driving home the point, I would not consider suggesting that you obtain your trace mineral chromium by licking your chrome bathroom fixtures. And I hope you would not consider doing so.

11. Scientists know a lot about the substances in real foods, but they certainly don't yet know all the substances that exist in foods. They continue to discover new (to them) nutrients and substances all the time. This means that, unless you are taking real food concentrates as supplements, you are not getting everything you need. You're being cheated. And your body knows.

12. The more a food is purified or a vitamin complex is purified or artificially copied, the *less nutritious* it becomes.

13. No one knows exactly what amounts and what mixtures of separated nutrients are best for health. Further, no one knows what amounts of mixtures of separated nutrients are best for you as a unique individual. Foods and food concentrates allow your body to *choose* what it needs in the amounts it needs at that particular time (it's called selective absorption).

14. Separated and/or synthetic nutrients create *imbalances* in your biochemistry. Attempts to "maximize" (single-out or imitate) one component from a food affects the accumulation or reduction of other components in your body. Taking large amounts of even several separated components can still result in "unexpected metabolic interactions within the body." In other words, while you're trying to correct one deficiency, you may be creating more problems in other areas of your biochemistry and body. Imbalances can be worse than deficiencies.

15. Individual vitamins or other isolated nutrients have pharmacological, *drug-like*, actions and will stimulate or suppress some segment of metabolism or a biochemical reaction. Thus, even though taking an isolated nutrient may reduce or create symptoms, it is *not feeding* the body's cells as do real foods and *not* truly improving health to its optimum level. Only whole foods and whole food supplements can accomplish this. You can't fool Nature.

16. Separated, non-food, or artificially-copied nutrients, particularly if taken in large doses or for a long period of time, can create *side effects*. This is because the body does not recognize them as "food" and cannot use them as true nourishment, as natural nutrient complexes or networks. In fact, isolated or synthetic vitamins create what has been called "expensive urine"—the body dumps most of what has been taken in. This is because the body doesn't know the chemicals as food and treats them as alien, as toxins. As much of the chemicals as possible is rushed through the bloodstream to the kidneys where they are excreted. Not so with real food. The body knows it's food, takes from it all the nutrients it needs and can get, then excretes only the leftovers and fiber.

There are many, many complex interactions of bioactive substances in a food. A single chemical compound can't even come close to matching the intricate, interrelated, synergistic functions of real, whole foods. Vitamins, phytochemicals, minerals, and other substances don't act the same way when they are separate parts and inserted into foods as in "fortified" or "enriched" edibles. Relying on supplements made of chemical parts is really the opposite of real nutrition. When you take a vitamin, mineral, phytochemical, amino acid, or other substance out of a food, you are taking it out of the environment in which it is most effective, most nutritious. Nutrients don't work in vacuums—they interact and they're inter-related as complete packages. That's why foods are the best way to get them.

"But," you say, "isn't there a difference between 'essential' and 'non-essential' nutrients? Shouldn't I only need the essential ones which I can get in supplements that separate them out?" Essential nutrients are classified as essential because they can't be made in the body from scratch and, therefore, must be obtained from foods. What's wrong with taking supplements that simply contain the essential nutrients, to make sure we get them, without bothering with all the other ones which we probably (wishful thinking) will get from our diet or can conjure up in our bodies? For one thing, the distinction between essential and nonessential nutrients is inconsistent with the fact that people are all different, unique. You and I vary in our capacity to make, transport, metabolize, and store nutrients, as well as our ability to respond to challenges and stress. We each have different nutritional needs. For another thing, a nutrient might be essential under one set of circumstances, but nonessential under other conditions. An individual's body—assumed to be able to make a nutrient—may be unable to do so under particular circumstances. As Dr. Buck Levin, a registered dietician, emphasizes, "From a functional perspective, all nutrients would therefore be categorized as 'conditionally essential.'" We need them *all* and the only way to get them all is by a variety of real, natural, whole foods.

Have you ever grown vegetables or fruits in your own garden? Or have you ever visited an organic farm? Picking or pulling up a fresh food from the rich soil in which it is grown is a special experience that nourishes your very soul. There is something in you that just knows this is a good thing, that there is a connection between you and that real, fresh, naturally-grown food. Several supplement companies produce one, two, or several whole food supplements while the remaining products offered are made of isolated, imitation chemicals (sometimes in a small base of whole foods). Very few supplement companies grow their own organic foods to make their own food supplements. Standard Process, Inc is one of them. Many of its supplements consist of these real foods. Visiting its extensive organic farm and processing facility is awe-inspiring. I have witnessed the harvesting of beautiful, healthy plants like huge red beets, bright crisp carrots, green and purple kale, and Spanish Black radishes that are handled immediately so that they are transformed into supplements within a day. It is a transformative experience. You know these supplements have to make your body's cells smile with appreciation. What a contrast to visiting a supplement company that uses purified white chemicals shipped in from various manufacturers that are stored in big plastic barrels and used when needed to process them into hard little pills or capsules. A friend who toured such a supplement company complained of a chemical odor that permeated the factory. The fumes left him with a two-day headache. Such synthetic supplements will receive no smiles from your cells. They are just something your cells have to figure out what to do with. Your body needs real foods and real food supplements, not manufactured chemicals. Your body innately knows this truth. Now it's just a matter of letting it sink into your (possibly previously misled) mind.

"When I was working in Bangladesh," says Dr. Rhona MacDonald who campaigned for access to essential medicines, "I witnessed a certain drug company promote the virtues of a sugar-coated vitamin pill as the most important factor in helping children grow and stay healthy. Families spent a day's wages on these useless tablets when they could have been buying bananas, spinach, and dahl (a bean dish) instead. As I watched parents make sacrifices to pay for these pills, I realized that I was obliged to do something about this profoundly unjust situation: now that I knew what was going on, doing nothing would make me complicit in the drug company's actions."

I can't help finding myself getting angry when I read things like this. What about you? Are you falling for commercial promotions by spending money on "useless tablets" of fabricated so-called nutrients when you could be getting real, natural foods and real, natural-food supplements?

References:

Bauer, Joy, "Fruity Snacks," *Self*, June 2007: 119.

Buhner, Stephen Harrod, *The Lost Language of Plants*, White River Junction, VT: Chelsea Green Publishing, 2002: 45-50, 145-150.

Lee, John R, "There's a Fuzzy Side to Nutritional Science," *The John R Lee, MD, Medical Letter*, Sept./Oct. 2001: 1-3.

Buhner, Stephen Harrod, *The Secret Teachings of Plants*, Rochester, VT: Bear & Company, 2004: 22-48.

DeCava, Judith A., *The Real Truth About Vitamins and Antioxidants*, Ft Collins, CO,:Selene River Press, 1995/2006.

Finley, John W., et al "Interactions Between Selenium and Secondary Plant Compounds," *Journal of Nutrition*, May 2005: 135(5):1236-1238.

Hite, Stuart, "Whole Foods vs. Isolated Nutrients," *HealthKeepers*, Spring 2005: 7(2):22-23.

Jacobs, David R., and Linda C. Tapsell, "Food, Not Nutrients, Is the Fundamental Unit in Nutrition," *Nutrition Reviews*, Oct. 2007: 65(10), 439-450.

Levin, Buck, *Environmental Nutrition*, Vashon Island, WA: HingePin Integrative Learning Materials, 1999: 16-113.

Macdonald, Rhona, "Access to Essential Medicines and the Pendulum of Power," *The Lancet*, 24 Mar. 2007: 369(9566), 983-984.

Minten, William, "The Real Secret," *Ode*, Jan./Feb. 2008: 6(1):15.

Pizzorno, Joseph, "Synthetic or Natural—Which Supplements Are Best?," *Integrative Medicine*, Dec. 2005/Jan. 2006: 4(6):6-8.

Pollan, Michael, *In Defense of Food*, New York, The Penguin Press, 2008.

Rice, Monica, "Whole Foods Are the Key To Good Health," *Spirituality & Health*, Mar./Apr. 2008: 11(2):30.

Scianna, Mary, "Vitamin Supplements: Good for Children?," *Today's Parent*, June 2006: 45.

Wieringa, F.T., J. Berger, et al, "Combined Iron and Zinc Supplementation in Infants Improved Iron and Zinc Status, but Interactions Reduced Efficacy in a Multicountry Trial in Southeast Asia," *Journal of Nutrition*, 2007: 137(2): 466-471.

FOOD FOR THOUGHT

"The Vitamin C antioxidant power of 8 oranges in 1 Nature Made tablet," reads the ad. Oh really? If you eat 5 to 10 servings of fresh fruits and vegetables a day, you should easily get the recommended 75 to 90 milligrams of vitamin C you minimally need. The "vitamin C" tablets like those in the ad are nothing more than ascorbic acid, in this case 500 milligrams per tablet. It doesn't replace real food—not by a long-shot. A real orange, for example, contains the entire vitamin C network which includes flavonoids, rutin, copper, and other components as well as some calcium, potassium, vitamin B_1, carotenes, folate, fiber, and all sorts of phytochemicals that aren't in the ascorbic acid pills.
Reference: Nutrition Action Healthletter, Oct. 2006: 9.

Food provides nutrients or "fuel" to cells so they can function properly. *Drugs* change or modify functions—they force, stimulate or suppress something. Food and drugs are totally different. Why on earth would we want to change foods so they behave like drugs?

As folks get older, the ability to produce hydrochloric acid in their stomachs may decrease and they may not digest some foods or absorb some nutrients, like calcium, the way they used to. To me, one of the worst things they can do is take Tums® or something like it to get their calcium. Antacids do away with hydrochloric acid, making it even more difficult to absorb calcium. And we can't expect older people,—or younger people—to absorb the calcium from oyster shells or coral, the contents of some calcium supplements.

Vitamins, phytochemicals (plant components), and other ingredients of real foods "don't act the same way when they are isolated and inserted into food," says Joy Bauer, RD. Real foods have so many biologically-active compounds that it is absolutely impossible to duplicate all their ingredients or inter-relationships in packaged goods or imitation supplements.
Reference: Bauer, Joy, "'Fruity' Snacks," *Self*, June 2007: 19(6):119.

French researchers reported that *each* vegetable or fruit serving you add to your day may reduce your risk of heart disease by as much as 7%. For a long time, research has linked the consumption of plenty of fruits and vegetables to a lowered risk of heart disease. Scientists have many theories for how these foods are protective, but so far, they haven't been able to identify "the" ingredient or ingredients that work the magic. "Possibly, there are synergistic effects..." offers dietician Tara Gidus, a spokesperson for the American Dietetic Association. People like Dr. Royal Lee said that there was synergy some 75 years ago. I've been saying that for, well, I won't say for how many years.
Reference: "Love that Produce!," *Eating Well*, Jan./Feb. 2007: 6(1):37.

Some minerals are known to be absorbed from foods as "components of complex organic entities"—whole packages—not just as separate chemicals that may be called "minerals."

Reference: Schzuss, Alexander G., *Minerals, Trace Elements and Human Health,* Tacoma WA: Life Sciences Press, 1996: 15.

Natural nutrient complexes in real foods are found in organic combination with each other—vitamins, minerals, trace minerals, enzymes, coenzymes, and other cofactors—that are not all present in separated or crystalline-pure or imitation preparations. When you separate the components, according to Dr. Royal Lee, you destroy the "biological relation and value." You break up the team. No chemist can reproduce or imitate nutrient complexes from real foods. "Just as the chemist cannot create life, neither can he create a complex vitamin: the life element in foods and nutrition. This is a mystery the chemist has never solved and probably never will, and the synthetic vitamins he creates on the basis of chemical formulae bear as much resemblance to the real thing as a robot does to a living man, lacking an elusive quality that chemistry cannot supply."

Reference: Lectures of Dr. Royal Lee, Volume 1, Fort Collins CO: Selene River Press, 1998: 158.

"We know today,"said Dr Royal Lee in a lecture in 1943,"that beriberi cannot be cured with synthetic vitamin B, and that scurvy cannot be cured with synthetic vitamin C. They are only relieved to some degree; to afford a cure, the complete natural vitamin complex is necessary. Still, the makers of these products are permitted to call them vitamins." Nowadays, it is not uncommon to see patients or clients with subclinical (not strikingly conspicuous) scurvy and beriberi. Synthetic vitamin C (as ascorbic acid) and separated synthetic B_1 will not cure these less-obvious problems either. We need the real deal, the intact pack.

Reference: Lectures of Dr. Royal Lee, Volume 1, Fort Collins CO: Selene River Press, 1998: 30.

"When you eat natural foods," explained Dr Royal Lee, "you get nature's complete prescription without any need on your part for selection." He would often repeat the point that most nutritional problems "come from the fact that we are trying to make something out of nothing." Unfortunately, there is now more effort to make something out of more nothing.

Reference: Lee, Royal, lecture, "Food Integrity," Apr. 1955: 4, 17.

When lecturing, Dr. Royal Lee would instantly begin to glow when asked about the difference between natural and synthetic vitamins. "Well, I'm glad that question came up. One is a chemical and one is a living thing..." he would begin. Then he would hold his audience in awe as he explained the stark differences. Natural food nutrients are complexes composed of known and unknown factors (to this day, some are still unknown). Separated or imitation nutrients may "fool a lot of people," but eventually some missing factor will make itself known "by the failure of the product to supply the expected nutritional action, by its failure to create health."

Reference: Lee, Royal, lecture, "Food Integrity," Apr. 1955: 37, and "Malnutrition As a Primary Cause of Disease," 23-24 Oct. 1943: 5.

An inorganic, nonfood mineral is as much different from an organic, food mineral "as a lump of brass is different from a watch," explained Dr. Royal Lee. "One is organized to perform a specific function, the other is not." Don't buy cheap imitations. Get the real thing.

Reference: Lee, Royal, lecture, "Food and Its Function," Coronado, CA, 12-15 Apr. 1951.

Want to start your own supplement company? There are oodles of manufacturers who will sell you just about any chemical "nutrient" formulation in bulk at wholesale prices—just check the Internet. You won't need a license. The most difficult part is how to make your pills appear to be better than the plethora of other supplements on the market. That's where marketing and advertising comes in:

"Doctor Recommended." Instant credibility. If you can't find a real MD, then you can get a photo of a competent-looking person in a white lab coat with a stethoscope draped around his or her neck. *"Doctor strength."* What does this mean? More drug-like chemicals? *"FDA approved laboratory"* is meaningless and false but does imply that the supplements are FDA-approved when they aren't. Similarly, *" FDA regulated"* is meaningless since, at this time, supplements are only very loosely regulated. The manufacturer is responsible for ensuring that its products are safe; and no laws require manufacturers to prove that their products actually work. *"Recommended by pharmacists."* Pharmacists are educated about drugs, not nutrition or food. Think about it. Also consider, for example, that GNC has been the business partner of Rite-Aid since 1999. It wouldn't be a hard endorsement for GNC-brand supplements to get. *"Patented."* This costs a little time and money, but getting a patent for your pills means big bucks. You don't even have to prove that your supplement works. *"Clinical studies."* Another sales booster. If your supplement is "clinically proven" to do something, it has to sell, right? Trouble is, even if your pills don't work really well, you can still boast about them. *"World's most powerful."* If you say so. Also good is *"no other supplement of this kind works better,"* maybe because all the other supplements of that kind are just as mediocre. The fact is that most supplements don't do what their makers imply by advertising. A measly few shreds of evidence and a supplement company may imply that it can prevent or treat some condition or disease. The Food and Drug Administration (FDA) can jump on a blatant lie, but subtle implications and lead-ons are harder to legally nail down.

Not all supplements are worthless or potentially harmful, of course. Real natural food supplements deliver the real whole food package that your body can use beneficially. But you should know where your supplements come from, exactly what is in them, and how they are processed. If you can't figure it out, enlist the aid of a competent nutritionally-savvy health professional.

References: Schardt, David, "The World's Most Powerful Doctor-Recommended Pat-

ented Now Available Without a Prescription As-Seen-On-TV Supplement," *Nutrition Action Healthletter*, Sept. 2007: 34(7), 9-11.
"Ask the Experts," *UC Berkeley Wellness Letter*, Oct. 2007: 24(1), 7.

Pharmaceutical companies now spend $4.5 billion a year just to advertise drugs directly to consumers. (This doesn't include all the ads and sales pitches to doctors via medical journals and office calls.) How many ads do you see on TV? From 2005 to mid-2006, drug companies spent $155 million to lobby members of Congress.
Reference: Health & Healing, Mar. 2007: 17(3), 5 & June 2007: 17(6), 5.

Pharmaceutical companies make far more money than supplement companies. One of the biggest means of cashing in is by formulating new drugs promoted as remarkable advancements. All too often, older, less expensive drugs are just as "good." Out of the 569 new drugs approved by the FDA from 1995 to 2000, only 13% contained new ingredients or were significantly better than older drugs. Yet the price tags were and are high, chokingly high. And doctors "educated" by the drug detailers (sales people) prescribe them.

How about all the scientific research that goes into producing drugs? It used to be that medical research was university-based and publicly funded. Nowadays, most of it is performed by for-profit organizations funded by drug companies. "Either a study is designed to maximize sales or it is designed to determine the best way to prevent or treat a particular health problem," explains John Abramson, MD, in his book, *Overdosed America*. Either sales or helping a health problem—you can't have it both ways. Guess which usually wins out? About 75% of the clinical studies in the top medical journals are commercially-funded. Studies that have negative results (showing the drug being tested is ineffective) are less likely to get published than studies with positive results (showing benefits). Results are frequently manipulated, harmful side effects are covered up, and scientific standards are overlooked. The idea is to sell drugs.
References: Abramson, John, *Overdosed America*, HarperCollins, 2004.
Whitaker, Julian, *Health & Healing*, June 2006: 16(6), 1-3.

Are North Americans getting healthier and living longer? The US World Health Report for 2001 showed that the life expectancy of people in most countries was between 71 and 73 years at a healthcare cost of $2,000 to $3,000. A couple of countries outside the average were the Czech Republic with a life expectancy just over 68 years at a cost of $1,000, and Japan's life expectancy of 75 years at a cost of $2,000. The US came in at just over 68 years with a cost of more than $5,000. Medical care costs in this country are 100% above the world average and we have a life expectancy under the world average. According to researchers at Johns Hopkins, "on most health indicators, US relative performance has declined since 1960; on none did it improve." Message: you must take more responsibility for your own health.
Reference: Martin, Paul, Gerson Healing Newsletter, May/June 2005: 20(3), 6.

A poll of Harvard University doctors (MDs, PhDs) and researchers showed that nearly three out of four eat fewer than five daily servings of fruits and vegetables, nearly half exercise only two times a week or less, and—are you ready?—about half call themselves enthusiastic, open-minded, or curious about alternative medicine. What about "physician, heal thyself?"

Reference: Martin, Adam, "Who's Healthier—You or Your Doctor?," *Health*, Apr. 2006: 20(3), 92.

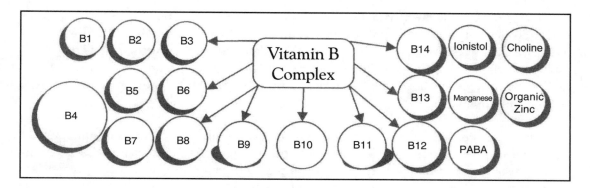

WHAT DO WE KNOW?

Scientists have discovered a tremendous amount of information about the contents, the ingredients, of foods. This includes, of course, nutrients. I remember, years ago, scientists saying that they had identified all of the nutrients in foods. They knew it all. Then they began to find phytonutrients, plant chemicals or nutrients. Since then thousands of phytonutrients have been identified. And more substances continue to be found. The truth is, we simply don't know everything about food or nutrition. There are components, relationships, activities, affiliations, and collaborations in real foods and real nutrient complexes that science has not yet uncovered.

Sometimes, from how people respond to foods and nutrient complexes, we can surmise, or guess, at some of the ingredients or their activities. Take B vitamins, for example. According to most nutritional charts, the B vitamins are thiamin (B_1), riboflavin (B_2), niacinamide (B_3), pyridoxine (B_6), biotin (B_7), folate (folic acid in imitation form), and B_{12}. Yet some really intelligent people have deduced that there is much more to the B-vitamin story. Choline, inositol, pantothenic acid, pangamic acid (called vitamin B_{15}) and para-aminobenzoic acid always appear as associates of the above B vitamins. Many of us consider them part of the vitamin B complex. Manganese, zinc and other minerals and trace minerals come with B vitamins in foods and evidently (even from scientific research) are essential to the overall function or activation of B vitamins. They should be part of the B complex too. So should some proteins and enzymes with the amino acids they contain. Then there are substances, such as one once identified as vitamin B_4, that have been discounted by scientists but exert a definite influence on people's biochemistry that cannot be totally explained by the action of the B vitamins accepted in scientific circles.

There are more questions. Here's one. B vitamins are categorized as "water-soluble." This means they dissolve in water and are harmed or destroyed by heat such as that used in cooking. On the other hand, "fat-soluble" vitamins are not as affected by temperature and are largely retained when foods are cooked. Now explain this: In countries that depend on rice for a large portion of their diet, people who eat refined rice develop nerve-related problems due to deficiencies of B vitamins, whereas those who eat brown rice do not. The brown rice contains the germ which houses most of the B vitamins. Refined rice has had the germ removed and so the B vitamins are mostly absent. The people eating brown rice cook it. If the B vitamins, being water-soluble, are supposed to be depleted or destroyed by heat, then how are they benefiting from these B vitamins? Could it be that there are fat-soluble B vitamins? I think so. Scientists have already discovered a fat-soluble nutrient that closely resembles what they know of as thiamin (B_1). And the discredited B_4 has always been identified by the nutritional mavericks as fat-soluble. More needs to be discovered.

So how can we think that a pill containing one or several chemical parts or imitations of a nutrient can be the same as what we would get in a real, Nature-made, intricately intertwined, secrets-yet-to-be-discovered food complex? In some respects, then, perhaps we could think of B vitamins, as our example, of having many more parts, many more *numbers*, as pictured here. And there's a very good chance that there should be more numbers than we could fit in this illustration.

Chapter Eight

CHEMICALS VS. FOOD

Food is far more than the sum of its parts. Yet that's what scientists usually look at—parts. And they usually believe that parts concocted in a laboratory are the same as real nutrients. Not so. There are many examples that show the difference between nutrient parts or synthetics and whole, natural food networks. Thousands and thousands of examples are embodied as patients and clients of doctors, nutritionists, and other health professionals. Unfortunately, "clinical evidence" (what happens with real people in real life) is frequently not accepted as "proof" in scientific circles. Scientific studies are considered the standard, even though they are sometimes less than clear, skewed, or downright silly. Nevertheless, reality sometimes seeps through. Here are some examples of what rationally shows up in recent scientific studies:

Most of the 52% of North American adults who take multivitamins/minerals—made of chemical, nonfood, nutrient parts—probably assume that there is some solid scientific evidence proving these pills support their health. But there isn't. A report issued by a National Institutes of Health expert panel concluded: "The present evidence is insufficient to recommend either for or against the use of multivitamins/minerals by the American public to prevent chronic disease." And these types of supplements may have side effects. This applies not only to "high-potency" single-nutrient supplements, but also to consuming "fortified" foods in addition to multi-vitamin/mineral supplements. No side effects occur by eating untampered-with, real foods. There's plenty of solid evidence that real natural foods do have real health benefits.

A study suggested that men who take more than one multivitamin a day—and especially those who took "individual" supplements—separated and/or synthetic—such as beta-carotene, zinc, selenium and others, were more likely to develop problems like prostate cancer than men who didn't. These supplements consisted of isolated parts and, mostly, manufactured imitations. Real whole food nutrients do not disturb the body this way.

Clinical trials (supervised experiments on people) that tested separated or manufactured supplements—such as beta-carotene, certain B vitamins, vitamin E (as d-alpha-tocopherol), and others—"have failed to show reduced chronic disease risk, and in some cases have shown increased risk," as the National Institutes of Health report stated. Trying to figure out what goes wrong, researchers are admitting that the many cooperative substances in real foods may contain a lot more information about health than does the specific component that they focused on. Using an individual part means a lot of information is lost. And little, if any, health benefits are gained. It can actually cause more harm than good.

In a randomized trial of 1450 women, some were given ascorbic acid (a synthetic vitamin C part), so-called vitamin E (a separated part), and beta carotene (an imitation) and some were given a placebo. There was no real difference in cardiovascular disease between the two groups. There were "no overall effects of ascorbic acid, vitamin E, or beta carotene" among women at high risk for cardiovascular disease. But eating foods like fresh fruits and vegetables, rich in the whole vitamin C complex, whole vitamin E complex, and numerous carotenes—which all work together and with myriad other food components—are connected with reduced rates of cardiovascular disease. It was "pills versus produce" and produce won. What about the pills? It was concluded by the lead author, Nancy R Cook, ScD, that "widespread use of these individual agents for cardiovascular protection does not appear warranted." Stick to real food.

In 47 randomized trials that included almost 181,000 adults, researchers found that taking separated, usually synthetic, vitamins A, E and beta carotene alone or in combination may increase the risk of dying by up to 16%.

After research linked diets rich in beta-carotene with a reduced risk for cancer, scientists figured that separated or synthetic beta-carotene supplements might also help prevent cancer. But they didn't. Two large trials in the 1990s showed that taking mega-dose beta-carotene supplements increased rates of lung cancer in smokers. Another large study, in which very few participants were smokers, did not show any increase in cancer, but it didn't show any decreased risk either. Synthetic beta-carotene failed. On the other hand, beta-carotene as a component in real whole foods does not present any danger and the foods definitely show cancer-protecting effects. Nature doesn't isolate nutrient parts. They are always natural parts of huge cooperative consolidations.

Synthetic beta-carotene differs from naturally occurring beta-carotene. Thus, doctors like Alan R. Gaby, MD, insist that "the best way to consume beta-carotene is by eating fruits and vegetables, which contain a wide array of different carotenoids." Supplementing with beta-carotene by itself can deplete other carotenoids and other nutrients, causing imbalances. It has been found that too much beta-carotene leads to a complicated chemical process that actually destroys an active form of vitamin A (retinoic acid) that regulates cell function and which has anti-cancer properties.

Consuming lutein (another carotene) by itself as a supplement will decrease beta-carotene concentrations in the body. Eating foods like yellow carrots, rich in lutein, does not decrease beta-carotene concentrations.

Taking synthetic vitamin A (as retinyl palmitate) can result in decreased calcium absorption and disruption of normal bone metabolism. This chemical "vitamin A" has even been put into gumballs, food bars, and other nonfoods. Some diet and energy bars contain almost 32,500 IU (10,000 mcg), which is more than 16 times the recommended daily dietary intake.

Scientists from Harvard found that the risk of pancreatic cancer was reduced by 81%, 73%, and 59% if the diets (food) of people contained good amounts of vitamin B_6, B_{12}, and folate, respectively. *But,* if people were given supplements containing separated, manufactured versions of these nutrients, their risk was not reduced. The study showed that they may even have a slight increased risk.

Maybe you've heard that taking mega doses (400 milligrams a day) of riboflavin (vitamin B_2) might ease the pain of a migraine headache. Or that it prevents cataracts. Neither has been proved. And there is a lot of doubt that you'll benefit since it would perform more as a drug, not a nutrient. Clue: Your body eagerly clears "excess" riboflavin—it turns your urine fluorescent yellow. This doesn't occur when you eat foods that contain riboflavin. Answer: Your body quickly tries to get rid of a foreign chemical substance it does not recognize as food.

Megadoses of separated or synthetic vitamin B_6 can produce toxic nerve disorders and degeneration. Too much niacin—vitamin B_3, the manufactured version of which is often used in large doses to reduce blood levels of cholesterol—can damage your liver and irreversibly change how your body processes blood sugar. On the other hand, food sources of B vitamins are essential to—and support—nerve health, liver function, and blood sugar metabolism.

I can think of numerous cases wherein people experienced side effects by taking synthetic B vitamins or large amounts of one separated B vitamin. And, sadly, even though these vitamins would give them a "high" of sorts (a boost of energy, for example) they would subsequently lose the elation and think they needed more of the imitation vitamins. There was Steve who would get a quickened heart rate and nervousness from the B_1 he thought would relieve his fatigue. Marcia took a supplement of mixed synthetic B vitamins (not realizing they were synthetic), thinking it would help her depression. It did seem to lift her spirits for a while, but her depression continued and worsened. Reading that B_6 was good for edema, Jill took a substantial amount for quite a while. She developed tingling sensations in her hands and feet as well as mood swings. Jill had no idea this was connected to the B_6. In each case, supplying the total vitamin B package in food form not only seemed to alleviate the side effects, but the clients were amazed at how much better they began to feel. And remember, a diet high in refined sugars and other refined carbohydrates usually leads to a deficiency of B vitamins.

Folic acid is now known as one of the nutrients that prevents fetal neural tube defects. However, scientists confess that there is still some confusion regarding the extent to which the addition of synthetic folic acid to grain products reduced the incidence of neural tube defects in the United States. In scientific lingo, folic acid is a methyl donor. Since 1998, all commercial refined grain products in the US have been "fortified" with synthetic folic acid, which is also included in prenatal vitamins and in many multivitamin products that other people take. Yet, too much folic acid by itself can "overmethylate" genes, potentially causing great harm such as babies born with autism or other problems. Also, if folic acid concentrations in the body become too high, enzyme (catalyst) activities decrease. Real foods that naturally contain folate don't cause such imbalances or impairments.

The molecule labeled "folic acid" is rarely found in Nature. Plants actually make a number of very closely related molecules collectively, as a package, called "folate." But sometimes you will see "folic acid" and "folate" used interchangeably. Humans can sort of change folic acid into folates, but there's a lot about this that is not yet known. Research is now showing that methylfolate is a more active form in the body than folic acid. There's also a lot of evidence that vitamin B_{12} should be taken with any type of folic acid supplements. In other words, we should get folate in nutritional packages just the way Nature has produced them and wrapped them up for our well being.

Research reported in the October 2007 *British Journal of Nutrition* showed that folates (from real natural foods) are metabolized in the gut, whereas folic acid (separated imitation) is metabolized in the liver. Because the liver is easily saturated, fortifying flour with folic acid could easily lead to significant amounts of unmetabolized (unprocessed) folic acid floating around in the blood with a potential to cause any number of quandaries.

One problem with all the synthetic folic acid appearing in "fortified" grocery items relates especially to older people. As we have mentioned, nutrients always have close relationships with other nutrients. One nutrient connected with folic acid is vitamin B_{12}. As many people age, they don't absorb or process B_{12} as well as they used to and become deficient in B_{12}. Large amounts of folic acid can *mask* the early symptoms that warn of B_{12} deficiency. A recent study indicted that high levels of folic acid when there is a vitamin B_{12} deficiency actually *worsens* rather than masks anemia and cognitive symptoms. Left undetected, B_{12} deficiency can lead to irreversible nerve and brain damage. A study of 1,459 people over age 60 found that 25% were low in vitamin B_{12}, and they performed poorly on cognitive tests. Those who had excessive folic acid levels performed the worst, scoring about five times below people with normal levels. Some of the worst problems are seen in individuals who take supplements on top of eating folic-acid "enriched" foods. There are some breakfast cereals, for example, that are fortified with 400 micrograms (mcg) of folic acid—100% of the current daily recommendation—per serving. Many people eat more than the serving cited on the box. And they eat other "fortified" or "enriched" foods like commercial breads. And they take supplements with more folic acid. Some people get

1,000 mcg of folic acid just from breakfast alone. This is way too much of a synthetic chemical.

In pregnant women, a combination of high folic acid intake and low vitamin B_{12} status has been linked to an increased risk of insulin resistance (often a prelude to diabetes) and obesity in their children.

It's been reported that taking high amounts of *synthetic* folic acid can gradually cause metabolic problems, including reduced immune function and signs of cancer. Real natural foods rich in folates (whole nutritional packages) lessen the risks for cancers, but synthetic folic acid does not seem to reduce the risks. Instead, in large amounts, it could actually contribute to the risks.

Researchers in Norway found that supplementing 800 micrograms a day of synthetic folic acid was linked to a slight increase in heart attack risk.

Some scary research came from Tufts University. It found that the "fortification" of enriched grains with synthetic folic acid may possibly be contributing to an increase in colorectal cancer. Neural tube defects have decreased (although there is some question about synthetic folic acid contributing to miscarriage), but since the time that grain products were fortified with synthetic folic acid, there have been four to six additional cases of colorectal cancer for every 100,000 people each year compared to the years before. This increase is not explained by chance or by increased cancer screening. Other evidence indicates synthetic folic acid may increase breast cancer too. "The body's response to folic acid appears to be complex," says Joel Mason, MD. Indeed. Excess manufactured folic acid might accelerate the development of cancer. However, much scientific evidence indicates that folate, the stuff in real food, protects against colorectal cancer, breast cancer, and other cancers.

Hints that there was a problem with separated synthetic folic acid showed up in the 1940s when scientist Sidney Farber gave high doses to leukemia patients. Instead of curbing the abnormal production of cancer cells, "he got a tremendous expansion of the leukemia cells." A study at Dartmouth School of Medicine indicated an increased risk of advanced adenomas in people who took synthetic folic acid. The fake folic acid may promote other cancers. If large quantities are taken by individuals with existing cancers, it could accelerate the cancers.

"There are several reasons why we may have inadvertently created the opposite effect with (synthetic) folic acid fortification," explains Dr. Mason. One reason is that, as the total amount of synthetic folic acid ingestion increases, the mechanism that converts it into the folate form the body can use (methyltetrahydrofolate—don't even try to pronounce it) can become overwhelmed. Your body tries to do something with this foreign chemical, but it can't handle an overload. The leftovers "might have detrimental effects, as it is not a natural form of the vitamin." The human body was supposed to get the real deal in real food, not a fake piece in refined nonfood. Dr. Mason says: "People shouldn't be concerned about foods—like leafy green vegetables—that are naturally rich in folate." Food truth.

Folic acid "fortification" of grain foods started in 1998. During the next decade, concentrations of folate in the blood increased in the US population, then decreased. People aren't eating less of the fortified foods. They probably can't convert it into a useful nutrient. And there is the distinct probability that getting large amounts of it results in decreased amounts of other nutrients that it uses while attempting the conversion. The prestigious medical journal, *The Lancet*, reported a case of a woman who had an allergic reaction (with anaphylaxis) three times after ingesting synthetic folic acid. The doctors writing about this case suggested that some suspected grain allergies may actually be an allergy to synthetic folic acid in the grain products. The woman had no trouble with folates in foods. Allergic reactions are likely to become more common now that grains are being "fortified" with this chemical vitamin imitation.

Does folic acid help reduce the risk of cardiovascular disease? The results of many studies are mixed and conflicting. Very often, supplementation with synthetic folic acid does not help at all. A look at 12 trials revealed that synthetic folic acid did not prevent heart disease, though it seemed to help lower stroke rates in only one study. Folates, with its partners in real food packages, help to prevent heart disease because nutrients work in concert with other nutrients. Furthermore, the causes of diseases like cardiovascular diseases, are multifactorial—there are many contributing factors including many nutritional deficiencies.

The use of multivitamins containing anywhere from two to 30 micrograms of synthetic vitamin B_{12} have been ineffective at normalizing the vitamin B_{12} status in older folks (who are often deficient in B_{12}). Seniors with low blood levels of B_{12} who are given up to 100 micrograms of synthetic B_{12} are only rarely helped, if at all.

Vitamin D is in the news a lot since it is being "discovered" to be an invaluable nutrient to just about every aspect of our health. So people are rushing out to get vitamin D supplements. However, most are isolated imitations. One such vitamin D supplement given to elderly people with osteoporosis upped their blood levels of vitamin D, but did nothing for their bone mineral density.

In its active form in the body, vitamin D (1,25-D or calcitriol) is actually a hormone. In supplements, it occurs in two different forms: vitamin D_2 (ergocalciferol) or vitamin D_3 (cholecalciferol). D_2 comes from non-animal sources, such as fungi, that are exposed to ultraviolet light to convert their sterols into this form of vitamin D. D_3 is usually derived from lanolin (a mixture of cholesterol and fatty acids) from sheep's wool. D_3 is also the form our skin produces when exposed to sunlight and is the natural form found in food such as fish liver oil. For many years it was thought that these two were interchangeable, both good. But now, with closer scrutiny, it's known that the D_3 form is more preferable, more "potent" and longer-acting in the body. Yet the D_2 form is still often used to fortify foods and is usually used in supplements, although this is beginning to change. Furthermore, there has been a long-standing fear of vitamin D toxicity from taking too much. Yet, the thing that had not been taken into account—the same thing that is usually not considered with virtually all nutrients—is the interaction, relationship, and balance of nutrients.

There is compelling evidence that vitamin D toxicity results from a relative deficiency of vitamins A and K complexes (and possibly vitamin E complex). In real foods, nutrients come in assembled combinations with many other nutrients. And they occur in a food form that the body can recognize, use and/or excrete, according to its own discretion. A wonderful source of vitamin D complex is cod liver oil, which also happens to be a terrific source of vitamin A complex. It all works together. In all the known cases of vitamin D toxicity where the dose given was intentional, the form used was vitamin D_2. Other reported cases involve accidental consumption of huge doses that were not intended to be consumed. So far, vitamin D_3 in supplements, has not been used or studied as extensively as vitamin D_2.

"Neither foods nor the nutrients within them," writes Chris Masterjohn, "are ever consumed alone; rather, they are consumed within the broader context of a diet that provides a full spectrum of nutrients, not all of which are substantially present in each individual food." Even the most readily available source of vitamin D—natural sunlight, from which the body makes vitamin D—can't be considered by itself, but must be seen within the context of a diet providing other nutrients (such as vitamins A and K) which interact with the vitamin D.

Supplements of vitamin D imitations often contain around 400 IU. People living in the tropics have always obtained between 4,000 and 10,000 IU per day from the sunshine. They don't have toxic reactions. And, evidence is mounting that such high amounts of vitamin D may actually protect them from diseases, including cardiovascular diseases, osteoporosis, and various cancers.

Fatty animal products and eggs provide small amounts of vitamin D, but seafood is the source of larger amounts. Mushrooms contain tiny amounts, though larger amounts appear in some obscure types.

For many years vitamin E was classified as d-alpha tocopherol, which is only one part of the vitamin E complex. Now it's known that taking a lot of d-alpha tocopherol lowers the amount of gamma-tocopherol, another important part. Alpha-tocopherol by itself has been flunking many scientific studies as far as helping conditions which are known to be prevented or relieved by vitamin-E-containing real foods. The alpha-part doesn't improve thinking ability for older folks, for instance, whereas vitamin E-rich real foods benefit cognition, lower risk for Alzheimer's disease, and have other gifts for brain and nerves. Vitamin E from real foods is linked to lower death rates from cancer, cardiovascular disease, and other causes. It helps maintain the immune system. These health benefits have not really been found when only d-alpha tocopherol in supplements is used.

While foods containing vitamin E packages have beneficial effects on factors that can cause cardiovascular disease (such as blood pressure, blood sugar metabolism, disturbed fat levels, etc.), supplements of d-alpha tocopherol have "no effect" on cardiovascular disease risk factors and don't lower the risk of other chronic diseases.

Individuals who took 600 IU of d-alpha tocopherol—erroneously called "vitamin E"—for 10 years or people who took 400 IU for seven years—did not experience any reduction in heart disease, stroke, or cancer rates. Worse still, there was a 13% increased risk of heart failure in those who already had cardiovascular disease or diabetes. One study showed that supplements in excess of 400 IU of d-alpha tocopherol (the separated part) seemed to increase the overall risk of dying. A 2007 study found that d-alpha tocopherol did not help the thickness of arteries; it didn't help to relax and open the blood vessels, something important to prevent cardiovascular problems. Another study with head and neck cancer patients showed a 38% increase in all-cause mortality in those given 400 IU dl-alpha-tocopherol per day.

One lady, under the direction of her husband, was taking huge amounts of d-alpha tocopherol, a separated part of the vitamin E complex. She had been experiencing leg cramps and this vitamin fraction appeared to alleviate them. It was explained to both of them that this was probably because the alpha-tocopherol was causing calcium to leach from her bones into the muscles, thus easing the muscle cramping. But this was not treating the cause. And it was suggested that continuing the alpha-tocopherol could lead to more complications since depleting the bones of calcium was not a good idea. The husband completely rebuffed the advice. He knew better. He kept her on the supplement. The next time I heard about this woman was several months later. She had been ice skating and fell. The bones in her leg shattered—not just broke. She would have problems with that leg for the rest of her life.

On the other hand, people with high intake of vitamin E—mostly from food—have substantially lower death rates from cancer, heart disease, and other diseases. Only 10% of subjects were taking supplements. Food protects. Manufactured nutrient parts don't. Keep in mind that vitamin E packages are found in foods with fat—like nuts, unrefined oils, whole grains. We definitely need some fats in our diets.

Scientists are finally admitting that vitamin E "is not one substance." But unfortunately, as the *UC Berkeley Wellness Letter* says, it's believed that it is only "eight related compounds." They point to four tocopherols and four tocotrienols. This is a wonderful advance in scientific thinking, but they still don't get the picture that there are even more ingredients in the vitamin E complex. They do concede that "vitamin E" supplements (of d-alpha tocopherol) have yielded disappointing results in studies. "A healthy diet is a better way to get E," they tell us. Real foods—like nuts, seeds, green leafy vegetables, whole grains, and others—are best.

Taking supplements of only d-alpha tocopherol lowers gamma tocopherol in the body. Gamma tocopherol is being found to be extremely important in many ways. Tocotrienols have also been found to do many things for our health that d-alpha tocopherol doesn't. For example, they help balance cholesterol levels, are involved in inflammation and repair processes, support the health and integrity of blood vessel walls, and even aid in lowering elevated triglycerides (involved in insulin resistance and heart disease). Taking lots of d-alpha tocopherol by itself can imbalance the other tocopherols and the tocotrienols and the other members of the vitamin E complex.

In 1960 it was found that selenium had to have vitamin E in order to work. In fact, selenium has always been an integral part of the vitamin E network in real foods. Selenium is the trace element activator of the rest of the vitamin E complex. It all works together, not separately.

Vitamin C from foods, but not from the so-called vitamin C in most supplements—which is only synthetic ascorbic acid—is associated with a 50% reduction in oral pre-cancer risk. The synthetic vitamin showed no protection at all. Imitation carotenes and vitamin A showed no protection either. Studies consistently show that diets (real foods) rich in nutrients such as vitamin C complex, vitamin E complex, carotenes, vitamin A complex, and others are associated with reduced risk for chronic diseases such as respiratory diseases, cancer, stroke, and heart disease. Studies using single, often manufactured versions, have been ambiguous, contradictory, or disappointing. Various studies have indicated that such supplements may actually increase the risk of some problems.

A review of 30 studies that looked at synthetic vitamin C (isolated and manufactured ascorbic acid) did somewhat reduce the number of colds in people exposed to extreme physical stress, such as marathon runners. But for the general population, it doesn't seem to help prevent colds. Actually, it acts more as an antihistamine (a drug-like substance), not as a real nutrient complex. The athletes, no doubt, received the antihistamine effect. A study reported in January 2008 found that supplementing with ascorbic acid decreases training efficiency in people who exercise regularly. Evidently it prevents some cellular adaptations to exercise. Ascorbic acid has relatively poor intestinal absorption. It is quickly excreted from the body (a clue that the body does not recognize it as food and cannot use it as food), and it is instable.

Ascorbic acid is referred to as "vitamin C," yet it is never found in foods by itself—it is always a part of a nutrient complex (vitamin C complex)—and the ascorbic acid in supplements is virtually always a manufactured chemical derived from corn syrup. It is about as far from natural food as you can get. Claims that it will "knock out" a cold or flu are based on the fact that ascorbic acid (synthetic, by itself) performs as an antihistamine—a drug. Research has shown that ascorbic acid lowers blood histamine levels and reduces histamine release from white blood cells called mast cells. The body uses histamine in the wonderful natural process of inflammation and repair. An antihistamine (meaning "against histamine") works as a drug, suppressing the natural histamine. This is why ascorbic acid will sometimes reduce symptoms of a cold, for example, but *only* at a certain stage of the inflammation and repair process. In other words, it interferes with one or two stages of inflammation. Thus, complete repair may not take place.

A high intake of the so-called vitamin C as ascorbic acid, the manufactured imitation part, has been connected with an increased risk of death from cardiovascular disease in some people. On the other hand, vitamin C food packages are essential to help prevent and repair cardiovascular disease. So far, studies have not found that ascorbic acid helps with inflammation, but when the whole, natural vitamin C package is obtained from real foods like fruits and vegetables, it does indeed help inflammation processes.

People who ate the least amount of vitamin C-rich fruits and vegetables were three times as likely to develop arthritis. Those who ate the most vitamin-C rich foods appeared to be much better protected from arthritis.

Vitamin C from food—but *not* synthetic ascorbic acid supplements—may reduce the risk of oral cancer by almost 50%. This finding had scientists scratching their heads. They said that synthetic and natural ascorbic acid are "chemically identical." They couldn't see beyond their myopic mindset that foods are very different from inert imitation chemicals. Foods work.

Taking 1000 milligrams (1 gram) of synthetic ascorbic acid twice a day increased the risk for developing kidney stones. Three other recent studies found the same problem with ascorbic acid. But there is no evidence that vitamin C complex from food does this. Rather, it helps prevent them.

Camu-camu is an Amazonian fruit that is a very rich source of vitamin C complex, including its ascorbic acid segment. In a study involving male smokers (smoking depletes vitamin C from the body), one group was given camu-camu juice while another group was given separated synthetic ascorbic acid. Both groups were getting 1,050 milligrams of ascorbic acid except those who got the fruit juice got all the other natural parts of the vitamin C complex along with it. The people consuming the camu-camu juice ended up with much lower levels of substances used to measure tissue stress or damage. Those getting the ascorbic acid chemical did not experience such reductions. The researchers concluded that the protective effects of camu-camu juice "may be due to the existence of unknown" substances besides the ascorbic acid or "unknown" substances that help the function of the ascorbic acid. It's the whole food gift.

The adrenal glands (also called the "stress glands") require plenty of vitamin C complex. I can recall many examples of people, especially women, who had various signs of adrenal fatigue, such as chronic tiredness, low blood pressure, craving for salt and/or chocolate, depression, mood swings, and others. One lady, for instance, had been taking two grams (2000 milligrams) of ascorbic acid each day and had all of these, as well as other, symptoms pointing to adrenal exhaustion. Getting dressed in the morning was a major undertaking. Everything appeared to be overwhelming and stressful. She had no clue that the ascorbic acid was actually creating a deficit of tyrosinase, a copper-containing enzyme, and other components of the whole vitamin C complex that were essential to adrenal health. Supplying the vitamin C food package in supplements and in her diet, along with some other adrenal support, made her think she was reborn.

Some vitamins and minerals and many plant nutrients are called *antioxidants*. Since people who eat foods containing antioxidants benefit in numerous ways from them, it has been assumed that antioxidants are "the" answer to so many problems. Well, it hasn't turned out that way. Antioxidants by themselves have not been shown to reduce risk of cardiovascular disease or cancer, for example, whereas foods containing antioxidants do help. In some cases, the separated antioxidant parts appear to increase symptoms or risk. Very often, synthetic forms of antioxidants are used in studies and marketed supplements. These can have a different chemical structure or be used quite differently in the body from those in real foods. The synthetics can cause things to go awry. As Professor Alice H. Lichtenstein, DSc, sums it up, "There is evidence that high doses of individual nutrients previously thought to be protective can have adverse consequences." Instead, she recommends that we make better choices while shopping for food. Antioxidants in foods work synergistically with other components in food—the effect is much, much stronger, and beneficial, when all ingredients are present. In fact, antioxidants (meaning "against oxygen") seem to serve as factors that protect other functional nutritional constituents from oxidation or premature breakdown.

Some insightful scientists are realizing that antioxidants in food serve as indicators or markers of a host of ingredients that protect us against diseases. They are only a small part of the whole package. Thus, nutritionist Ronald Prior, PhD, points out that the total antioxidant capacity of a food does not necessarily reflect its potential health benefit. It's the whole food that benefits.

How about minerals? Mineral supplements can contain three forms. Usually they contain the least absorbable form—metallic. Rust, or iron oxide, is a metallic form of iron, for example. But it's not the form that appears in real foods that we are designed to eat. At best, metallic minerals are 10% absorbable, or "bioavailable," to our bodies at the cellular level. At least 90% pass right through our digestive tract.

During the 1960s, chelated minerals came on the scene. By attaching an amino acid to the clay or metallic form of a mineral, the absorption rate could be increased to 40 to 50%. The third form is colloidal. Colloidal minerals are very different from the other two. Plants extract the "rock" minerals from the soil in their crude metallic form and transform them into colloidal minerals, the form Nature intended for animals and humans to consume.

Additionally, like all food nutrients, minerals work with, depend on, and are related to, many other minerals and other nutrients. Taking one mineral by itself not only won't work as well, but may cause some chaotic consequences in our bodies.

Calcium is important to so many things, including your bones and immune system. But if you take non-food versions, you can't stop taking them because you lose the "benefit." The benefits from foods don't stop abruptly like that. Calcium works with magnesium, potassium, and vitamin D, among other nutrients. Taking too much of any one of these can create a deficit or imbalance of the others. Too much calcium supplementation by itself can even inhibit iron and zinc absorption. The best source is real food where minerals come in complete packages.

A review of 17 studies showed that people who consistently took separated calcium supplements reduced their risk of bone fractures, *but* if they missed doses more than 20% of the time, they reduced the benefits by half. Real food doesn't work like that. Everyone knows that calcium is needed to prevent osteoporosis and disabling fractures. But in an analysis of 12 population studies, women who took calcium-alone supplements were 65% *more* likely to suffer a broken hip than women not taking such supplements. Yet no link was found between fractures and *total* calcium intake from supplements *plus* food. The message is that calcium, just like every other nutrient, does not work alone. Vitamin D, minerals like phosphorus and magnesium and boron and manganese and others, proteins, and other food components are needed as well.

Researchers who looked at 1,471 postmenopausal women observed that the women taking separated calcium had a 47% higher risk of having a heart attack, stroke, or sudden death than women who got placebos. Overall evidence is inconsistent. Yet we know that taking one isolated nutrient can create imbalances of other needed nutrients. Evidence of the benefits of real foods is consistent. The pharmaceutical (drug) industry did not agree with the points presented from this study. Of course not. Drug companies manufacture a big chunk of the supplements on the market.

Nan Kathryn Fuchs, PhD, says you "don't need to take high quantities of calcium supplements. You need to get more calcium from your diet." Or from real food supplements, if needed. Researchers at Washington University School of Medicine, St. Louis, studied almost 200 postmenopausal women. The women who got most of their calcium from supplements of the separated mineral had lower bone density than those who got most from real foods. The combination of a good diet and supplements resulted in the highest bone density. Calcium, like all nutrients, needs companion nutrients to work. Bones also need magnesium, boron, strontium, manganese, vitamin C complex, and much more.

Pregnant women given calcium carbonate (a non-food version) experienced no benefits to their breast-milk calcium concentrations or to the birth weight, growth, or bone mineral status of their babies. More than 2,800 children given calcium in various forms—but just calcium—experienced little or no effect on their bone density. Whereas calcium from foods appears to reduce body fat in overweight individuals, calcium supplements have no such effect.

Magnesium intake balances calcium and phosphorus; calcium intake balances magnesium and phosphorus. Too much separate calcium reduces magnesium. Too much separate magnesium from supplements reduces calcium. And it can cause diarrhea, nausea, cramps, muscle weakness, and heart problems. This does not happen with real foods.

Excessive intake of calcium might interfere with absorption and use of magnesium, as Veronica found out as she gradually became more irritable and weak, developing muscle cramps and insomnia. Wasn't calcium good for these things? Yes, but too much calcium can create a relative deficiency of magnesium, causing such symptoms. Foods balance. Individual separated nutrients imbalance.

Can you get too much potassium from real food? No. Separated potassium supplements, though, can be disruptive. Problems in the digestive system, even ulcers, or an irregular heartbeat are the most serious side effects and occur with prescription potassium preparations often given to people treated with certain diuretics. High-potassium foods are much better than potassium "medications" and provide lots of other beneficial nutrients and balancers.

Non-food iron given to non-anemic women during pregnancy could be harmful, especially with respect to high blood pressure and the likelihood of giving birth to a low-weight baby. Yet it's known that iron is extremely important during pregnancy, for both Mom and baby, for things like thinking ability, memory, and behavioral functions, among others. Some studies show that non-food iron does little more than improve blood test results. It gets in the blood, but it doesn't work in the tissues.

Taking too much iron by itself can alter manganese, chromium, copper, zinc, and other nutrient levels in your body. In real foods, iron comes in a collective form with other synergists such as vitamin C complex (an enhancer of iron absorption), copper, zinc, manganese, vitamins A and D, B vitamins, and more. For instance, a deficiency of vitamin A impairs iron metabolism. Protein and other factors in foods like red meat enhance iron absorption. Food provides the integrated ensemble.

People with iron-deficiency anemia may be given intravenous non-food iron. Acccording to Dr. Jerome L. Sullivan, this can cause "possible delayed risks" of not achieving satisfactory responses and the procedute "ignores potential long-term adverse effects of storage iron load on survival."

Take too much zinc by itself and you can create a relative deficit of copper because it interferes with the absorption of copper. This leads to a decrease in the essential activity of SOD (superoxide dismutase), the "super" enzyme needed by your immune system, for one thing. Too much zinc may weaken your immune system, have a negative effect on your urinary tract, affect the body's ability to absorb and store calcium and copper, and may eventually lead to a debilitating anemia. "Copper often is overlooked as an important nutrient when considering diets that promote cardiovascular health in humans," according to the USDA's Agricultural Research Service. Foods containing zinc, on the other hand, come packed with a plethora of other nutrients for balance and for interaction. For example, getting zinc in your food improves your vitamin A status since they both work together. When you eat real foods, your body has "selective absorption," the ability to choose how much of each nutrient it needs.

One young man, who was into body-building, took lots of separated zinc, thinking it would help prevent the colds he was susceptible to, and, since it might increase sperm count and sexual performance, he figured it would make him that much more "macho." Eventually, though, his blood pressure began to creep up, he had trouble concentrating, he was getting even more colds, and he experienced more muscle injuries after his workouts. Excess zinc had created a deficit of copper with the resultant problems. It took a while for us to get his mineral balance back to normal. He swore off high-potency, separated nutrients—a big accomplishment considering his previous mindset.

You can get too much copper as well if you get it from supplements of separated minerals. High copper levels have been linked to increased risk of cardiovascular disease and cognitive decline in older people. Most people don't get enough copper from their diets, but scientists at the University of California, Berkeley, advise that you shouldn't take high–potency formulas or copper supplements. Most supplements containing copper, like most supplements containing any minerals, are not food forms as whole food packages.

Did you know that your thyroid needs, not only iodine, but also selenium, and that these two trace minerals work together? Selenium also increases the concentration of zinc and iron in places where they are needed, and reduces potentially too high concentrations of iron in the liver. But selenium chelate supplements are inorganic—not a food form. The effectiveness in real bodies is best when selenium comes from real foods.

The Nutritional Prevention of Cancer Study, which started in 1983, found that taking separated selenium supplements (200 micrograms a day) did *not* lower the risk of squamous and basal cell skin cancers in 1,312 people who lived in areas of the Southeast where selenium intakes are often low. In 2003, the researchers reported a slight *increase* in squamous cell skin cancers. Separated selenium supplements did not protect against heart disease either. Yet foods rich in selenium have shown protective effects in regards to cancers, cardiovascular disease, and other health issues.

It came as a surprise to researchers, but a study reported in the *Annals of Internal Medicine* seemed to show that (separated) selenium supplements might actually increase the risk of type 2 diabetes. Previous evidence indicated that folks who get selenium in their diets had a reduced risk of diabetes as well as various cancers and other problems. As scientists at the University of California, Berkely put it: "The safest way to get selenium is from food, such as whole grains, nuts (notably Brazil nuts), and seafood." Selenium, like all nutrients, is one component in foods that works cooperatively with all the other components in ways we haven't even fathomed yet. Food sources can improve blood sugar metabolism, but high doses of separated selenium have effects that are "unclear" at best.

Chromium, very important to blood sugar processing, is part of the "glucose tolerance factor," a combination of substances in real food. Yet, separating this combination into parts has not revealed the secret of the glucose tolerance factor. There is potential harm in long-term use of isolated chromium supplements. Best recommendation from the scientists: get your chromium from food.

There is plenty of evidence that individual needs for specific nutrients can vary greatly. This means that each individual has individual mineral and trace mineral requirements as well as individual requirements of all other food factors. *The Earth's Gift to Medicine* by K-G Wensel, MD and R.J. Pataracchia, ND, is a reference book about minerals. It delves into the interconnections between minerals in our bodies. Too much of one can cause a deficiency of others. For example, too much zinc decreases copper and manganese. Deficiencies of minerals, such as calcium, can lead to absorption of toxic metals such as lead and cadmium. The authors consider a balanced mineral profile as conducive to health. Real food gives your body a choice for absorbing what it needs in the amounts it needs to achieve that balance.

Taking amino acids has become popular. Amino acids are the building blocks of protein. But taking one or two individual amino acids is not a great idea. This creates imbalances of other amino acids and other nutrients. Branched-chain amino acids (leucine, isoleucine, and valine) are essential, but taken alone for a long time, they can cause toxic reactions in the nervous system. Cysteine can be quite toxic when taken in mega amounts.

Arginine is being used a lot because, from it, nitric oxide is produced, a "vasodilator" (which relaxes or opens up blood vessels). So it's given to folks with high blood pressure, angina or other cardiovascular diseases. And arginine seems to stimulate the immune response in healthy people. Yet it doesn't help the stiffness or hardness of blood vessels and, when given in high doses, it may cause problems with the immune system. In one study published in the January 4, 2006 *Journal of the American Medical Association*, people who had a heart attack were either given arginine or a placebo. The trial was stopped early after several people from the arginine group died (whereas none died from the placebo group). Like all nutrients, amino acids relate with other amino acids and other nutrients. Taking high doses of a single nutrient usually depletes other nutrients. Taking lysine supplements, for instance, lowers arginine levels in your body, which can compromise your immune system. However, foods rich in lysine or arginine are safe and helpful.

Carnitine on its own in high amounts has been associated with body odor, nausea, vomiting, abdominal cramps, heartburn, gastritis, diarrhea, and seizures. Controversy surrounds the use of big doses of creatine, used by athletes and others wanting to enhance their performance, to increase muscle production. Weight gain is a side effect. And there are numerous concerns about its use. Reports of muscle cramping and gastrointestinal effects are common and there are case reports involving kidney dysfunction. Glutamine is important to many tissues such as those that line the intestines. But it can produce side effects when taken alone. It doesn't help intestinal health in folks with tissue injury and inflammation, and there have been cases where evidence of liver stress occurred.

Tryptophan was banned from the market for a while because of causing EMS (eosinophilia-myalgia syndrome). This was found to be due to contaminated batches from a Japanese manufacturer. However, as many as 5% of EMS cases were not traced to contaminated tryptophan, suggesting that tryptophan itself may (rarely) cause EMS . Known possible side effects also include nausea, headache, lightheadedness, and drowsiness. Even the popular 5-HTP (a compound made from tryptophan) can cause heartburn, stomach pain, belching, flatulence, nausea, vomiting, diarrhea, and loss of appetite.

Phenylalanine is a common ingredient in sugarless gum and other sugar-free foods as a component of aspartame (the artificial sweetener NutraSweet). Some nerve specialists believe that aspartame may disrupt your brain function by overstimulating your neurons. There is a risk of birth defects during pregnancy. And phenylalanine supplements might cause high blood pressure or increase the risk of stroke in certain people. Lysine is used for recurrent herpes breakouts. Diarrhea and abdominal pain have been reported with its use at 10 grams a day for five days. High doses have been reported to increase the risk for gallstones.

Many other examples could be cited. The point is that real food or food concentrates are the best way to get your nutrients. Taken by themselves as amputated parts or, worse still, as manufactured facsimiles, they can cause biochemical distortions in your body. Actually, to me, they are not really nutrients because they cannot feed or nourish the body in the way real foods produced by Nature can.

The Organic Consumers Association is now engaged in a campaign to stop fraudulent labeling of synthetic vitamins and supplements as "natural," and to educate consumers about the benefits of food-based nutrients. As things stand, the word "natural" on a bottle of supplements doesn't mean anything. It should mean something that's not artificial or abnormal. But the term is nevertheless used to describe artificial imitations of nutrients and abnormal bits of nutrient complexes.

No matter how hard you try to get all the nutrients you need from supplements containing isolated or synthetic versions, you can't mimic the combination, intricate balance, and function of whole foods. Neither do you get all the nutrients since more are being discovered all the time. When nutrients are obtained from whole foods, they produce a much stronger effect than do any of the individual, broken nutrients.

Whole food concentrate supplements may contain low or even tiny amounts of specific nutrients. But, because all the components work together, the effect is far greater than single parts. You might be used to looking for "high potency" supplements, thinking you will get more of a good thing. That's not the case, and you may be getting something that's not good. "Potency" refers to power, influence, or strength. Real foods and real food supplements have far more power, influence, and strength as far as your body is concerned. It's a symphony, not a solo.

Cornell food scientist Rui Hai Liu and his colleagues spent years studying more than 8,000 phytochemicals and other components found in fruits, vegetables, and whole grains. They found that, because these various compounds differ in their molecular size, polarity, and solubility, they produce a powerful natural combination that's more biologically available to the body's cells, organs, and tissues than any single nutrient. For example, one medium apple with only about six milligrams of vitamin C has enough other components to produce the antioxidant activity of 1500 milligrams of ascorbic acid from supplements. Plant chemicals in whole grains are bound in the cells walls and, until recently, were thought to be an indigestible part of the fiber. About 90% of these plant chemicals in whole wheat are bound, passing through the stomach and small intestines undigested. But, these phytochemicals are released further down by the microflora (intestinal bacteria) in the colon. These compounds have very potent and powerful properties than can profoundly affect colon health, among other things. Refined-grain products with added synthetic vitamins can't come close—they're digested long before they reach the colon. Nature knows best. "We still don't know all the compounds that are important or how they work together," says Dr. Liu. Eating real food, and if needed, taking real food supplements are the way to go. "There is no other way to get that much nutrition."

The advantages of consuming real foods cannot be reproduced by extracting some so-called "active ingredient" and taking it in isolation. We can't rely on extracted parts or manufactured imitation parts to give us what we need nutritionally. Research, and, may I add, the effects on actual human beings, has demonstrated that the benefits of real food are far more complex than merely delivering so many milligrams or micrograms of this or that vitamin, mineral, or other nutrient. As Alice H. Lichtenstein, DSc, and Robert M. Russell, MD, wrote in the *Journal of the American Medical Association*, "Other factors in food or the relative presence of some foods and the absence of other foods [nonfoods] are more important than the level of individual nutrients consumed." In other words, there's a lot more to food than the nutrients that can be identified in them. It's Nature's secret. Don't mess with it.

References:
Acres USA, Feb. 2008:38(2),10.
Albert, C.M., N.R. Cook., et al, "A Randomized Factorial Trial of Vitamins C and E and Beta Carotene in the Secondary Prevention of Cardiovascular Events in Women," *Archives of Internal Medicine,* 13-17 Aug. 2007: 167:1610-1618.
"AMA Knocks Synthetics," *Acres USA*, Nov. 2007: 37(11), 73.
Antinoro, Linda, "Trace Minerals You Can't Live Without; How to Get Enough," *Environmental Nutrition*, Nov. 2007: 30(11), 1-6.
"Antioxidant Vitamins: Review Finds Increase in Mortality," *HealthFacts*, Apr. 2007: 32(4), 1-3.

"Arginine Is Beneficial to Health, but Also Risky," *Environmental Nutrition*, July 2007: 30(7), 7.

"Ask the Experts," *UC Berkeley Wellness Letter*, " Aug. 2007: 23(11), 7.

Badmaev, Vladimir, Muhammed Majeed, and Richard A. Passwater, "Selenium: A Quest for Better Understanding," *Alternative Therapies*, July 1996: 2(4), 59-67.

Bairatl, I., "Antioxidant Vitamins Supplementation and Mortality: A Randomized Trial in Head and Neck Cancer Patients," *International Journal of Cancer*, 2006: 119, 2221-2224.

Baker, David H., "Comparative Species Utilization and Toxicity of Sulfur Amino Acids," *Journal of Nutrition*, June 2006: 136(6S),1670S-1675S.

"Balancing Risks, Benefits of Folic-acid Fortification," *Tufts University Health & Nutrition Letter*, Oct. 2007: 25(8), 1-2.

Bazzano, L.A., K. Reynolds, et al, "Effect of Folic Acid on Risk of Cardiovascular Diseases: A Meta-analysis of Randomized Controlled Trials," *Journal of the American Medical Association*, 13 Dec. 2006: 296(22), 2720-2726.

Berger, A., H. Schaumburg, et al, "Dose Response, Coasting, and Differential Fiber Vulnerability in Human Toxic Neuropathy," *Neurology*, 1992: 42:1367-1370.

Berkoff, Nancy D., "Drink Milk or Bask in the Sun: Which Is Better for Vitamin D?," *Vegetarian Times*, July/Aug. 2007: 351, 23-24.

Bjelakovic, Goran, Dimitrinka Nikolova, et al, "Antioxidant Supplements for Prevention of Gastrointestinal Cancers: A Systematic Review and Meta-analysis," *The Lancet*, 2 Oct. 2004: 364(9441), 1219-1228.

Bjeladovic, Goran, Dimitrinka Nikolova, et al, "Mortality in Randomized Trials of Antioxidant Supplements for Primary and Secondary Prevention," *Journal of the American Medical Association*, 28 Feb. 2007: 297(8), 842-857.

Bliss, Rosalie Marion, "When it Comes to Vitamins, More Is Not Always Better," Agricultural Research Service, USDA, 16 Nov. 2007: www.ars.usda.gov/ispr.

Boekholdt, S.M., and M.C. Meuwese, "Plasma Concentrations of Ascorbic Acid and C-reactive Protein, and Risk of Future Coronary Artery Disease, in Apparently Healthy Men and Women: The EPIC-Norfolk Prospective Population Study," *British Journal of Nutrition*, 2006: 96(3), 516-522.

Braun, Michelle and Connie M Weaver, "A Call To Evaluate the Impact of Calcium-Fortified Foods and Beverages," *Nutrition Today*, Jan./Feb. 2006: 41(1), 40-47.

Buchman, Alan L., "Glutamine: Commercially Essential or Conditionally Essential? A Critical Appraisal of the Human Data," *American Journal of Clinical Nutrition*, July 2001: 74(1), 25-32.

Bunout, Daniel, Gladys Barrera, et al, "Effect of a Nutritional Supplementation on Bone Health in Chilean Elderly Subjects with Femoral Osteoporosis," *Journal of the American College of Nutrition*, June 2006: 25(3), 170-177.

"Calcium Alone May Harm Bones; Add D and Phosphorus, Try Food First," *Environmental Nutrition*, Mar. 2008: 31(3), 7.

"Calcium: Making it Add Up," *UC Berkeley Wellness Letter*, Aug. 2006: 22(11), 4.

"Calcium Supplementation for Children Has Little Effect on Bone Density," *HealthFacts*, Dec. 2006: 31(12), 5.

"Calcium Supplements Still Have a Role," *Environmental Nutrition*, June 2006: 29(6), 1-2.

"Can Too Much Copper Be Harmful?," *UC Berkeley Wellness Letter*, Nov. 2007: 24(2), 7.

Casanueva, E., et al, "Weekly Iron as a Safe Alternative to Daily Supplementation for Nonanemic Pregnant Women," *Archives of Medical Research*, 2006: 37, 674-682.

Cleary, Alison J., "Zinc," *Eating Well*, Oct./Nov. 2005: 4(3), 22.

"Cold Fighters," *Consumer Magazines Digest*, Nov. 2004, 16(11), 4.

Cole, Bernard, John Baron, et al, "Folic Acid for the Prevention of Colorectal Adenomas," *Journal of the American Medical Association,*, 6 June 2007, 297(21), 2351-2359.

"Cracking the D-vitamin Code," *UC Berkeley Wellness Letter,* Aug. 2007: 23(11), 2-3.

Cronin, Joseph R., "The Chromium Controversy," *Alternative & Complementary Therapies*, Feb. 2004: 10(1), 39-42.

Dattilo, Anne M., and Stanley G Miguel, "Chromium in Health and Disease," *Nutrition Today*, July/Aug. 2003: 38(4), 121-133.

Davison, G., and M. Gleeson, "The Effect of 2 Weeks of Vitamin C Supplementation on Immunoendocrine Responses to 2.5 h Cycling Exercise in Man," *European Journal of Applied Physiology*, 10 May 2006.

Dean, Carolyn, "Chewing Gum Side Effect," *Natural Health,* Oct./Nov. 2002: 32(8), 44-45.

Devaraj, Sridevi, Rong Tang, et al, "Effect of High-dose A-tocopherol Supplementation on Biomarkers of Oxidative Stress and Inflammation and Carotid Atherosclerosis in Patients with Coronary Artery Disease," *The American Journal of Clinical Nutrition*, Nov. 2007: 86(5), 1392-1398.

Edmunds, J.E., et al, "Creatine Supplements Should Be Used with Caution and Supervision, if at All, in Individuals with Renal Insufficiency," *American Journal of Kidney Diseases*, 2001: 37(1), 73-78.

Evans, Joanna, "Fortification Folly," *What Doctors Don't Tell You*, Nov. 2007: 18(8),10.

"Fight Cancer and Heart Disease with Healthy Food, Not Antioxidant Pills," *Tufts University Health & Nutrition Letter*, Dec. 2004: 22(10), 7.

"Folic Acid: Too Much of a Good Thing? Food Folate to the Rescue," *Environmental Nutrition*, Mar. 2008: 31(3), 1, 6.

"For Heart-risk Women, Pills Don't Protect Like Produce," *Tufts University Health & Nutrition Letter*, Nov. 2007: 25(9):1-2.

Fuchs, Nan Kathryn, "Antioxidants Protect Against Disease—but Some Healthy Foods are Surprisingly Low in Them," *Women's Health Letter*, Nov. 2006: 12(11), 6-7.

Fuchs, Nan Kathryn, "Dietary Calcium vs. Supplements," *Women's Health Letter*, Dec. 2007: 13(12), 4-5.

Fuchs, Nan Kathryn, "Woman to Woman," *Women's Health Letter*, May 2002: 8(5), 8.

Gaby, Alan R., "Let Your Food Be Your Medicine," *Townsend Letter*, Nov. 2004: 256, 25.

Gaby, Alan R., "Do Antioxidants Kill People?," *Townsend Letter*, June 2007: 287, 141-142.

Gaby, Alan R., "L-arginine for Angina Pectoris," *Townsend Letter*, Nov. 1999, 196:19.

Gaby, Alan R., "Glutamine Supplementation Not Recommended for Crohn's Disease," *Townsend Letter*, Oct. 2001, 219:18-19, citing A.K. Akobeng, et al, "Glutamine Supplementation and Intestinal Permeability in Crohn's Disease," *Journal of Parenteral and Enteral Nutrition*, 2000: 24, 196.

Gao, Xiang, Antonio Martin, et al, "A-tocopherol Intake and Plasma Concentration of Hispanic and non-Hispanic White Elders Is Associated With Dietary Intake Pattern," *Journal of Nutrition*, Oct. 2006: 136(10), 2574-2579.

Gardner, Amanda, "Calcium Supplements Could Raise Heart Risks in Postmenopausal Women," *www.healthfinder.gov*, 15 Jan. 2008.

Geiger, Sylvia M., "Beta Carotene," *Eating Well*, Mar./Apr. 2007: 6(2):23.

Geiger, Sylvia M., "Why You Need Niacin," *Eating Well*, May/June 2007: 6(3), 23.

Geiger, Sylvia M., "Why You Need Riboflavin," *Eating Well*, Sept./Oct. 2007: 6(5):48.

Gomez-Cabrera, Mari Carmen, Elena Domenech, et al, "Oral Administration of Vitamin C Decreases Muscle Mitrochondrial Biogenesis and Hampers Training-induced Adaptations in Endurance Performance," *The American Journal of Clinical Nutrition*, Jan. 2008, 87(1):142-149.

Goran, et al, *Journal of the American Medical Association*, 28 Feb. 2007: 297:842-857.

Greenfield, Russell H., "Selenium Too Sweet? Supplementation and Type 2 DM," *Alternative Medicine Alert*, Oct. 2007: 10(10), 117-118.

HealthNews, Mar. 2005: 11(3):15.

Hemila, Harri, and Edgar R. Miller III, "Evidence-based Medicine and Vitamin E Supplementation," *American Journal of Clinical Nutrition*, July 2007: 86(1), 261-264.

Hendley, Joyce, "How Much Folate Do You Need?," *Eating Well*, July/Aug. 2007: 6(4), 43.

Hobbs, Suzanne Halva, "How Can I Get enough Iron?," *Vegetarian Times*, Mar. 2006: 339, 33-34.

Houghton, Lisa A. and Reinhold Vieth, "The Case Against Ergocalciferol (vitamin D_2) as a Vitamin Supplement," *American Journal of Clinical Nutrition*, Oct. 2006: 84(4), 694-697.

Hughes, Suzanne, Samir Samman, et al, "The Effect of Zinc Supplementation in Humans on Plasma Lipids, Antioxidant Status and Thrombogenesis," *Journal of the American College of Nutrition*, Aug. 2006: 25(4), 285-291.

Hurrell, Richard F., Manju B. Reddy, et al, "Meat Protein Fractions Enhance Nonheme Iron Absorption in Humans," *Journal of Nutrition*, Nov. 2006: 136(11), 2808-2812.

Hutson, Susan M., Andrew J. Sweatt, et al, "Branched-chain Amino Acid Metabolism: Implications for Establishing Safe Intakes," *Journal of Nutrition*, June 2005: 135(6), 1557S-1564S.

Inoue T., H. Komoda, et al, "Tropical Fruit Camu-Camu (Myrciaria Dubia) Has Anti-Oxidative And Anti-Inflammatory Properties," *Journal of Cardiology*, 2008: 52(2):127-32.

"If Copper Is To Be Used, in What Amounts?," *Tufts University Health & Nutrition Letter*, Dec. 2007: 25(10), 7.

Jacobs, David R., Jr., and Linda C. Tapsell, "Food, Not Nutrients, Is the Fundamental Unit in Nutrition," *Nutrition Reviews*, Oct. 2007: 65(10):439-450.

Jaret, Peter, "Selenium," *Eating Well*, Aug./Sept. 2006: 5(4):20.

Jarjou, Landing M. A., Ann Prentice, et al, "Randomized, Placebo-controlled, Calcium Supplementation Study in Pregnant Gambian Women: Effects on Breast-milk Calcium Concentrations and Infant Birth Weight, Growth, and Bone Mineral Accretion in the First Year of Life," *American Journal of Clinical Nutrition*, Mar. 2006: 83(3), 657-666.

Johnson, A.R., A. Munoz, et al, "High Dose Zinc Increases Hospital Admissions Due To Genitourinary Complications," *Journal of Urology*, 2007: 177(2), 639-643.

Johnson, Mary Ann, "If High Folic Acid Aggravates Vitamin B_{12} Deficiency, What Should Be Done About It?," *Nutrition Reviews*, Oct. 2007: 65(10), 451-458.

Jones, Vaughan, "The Power of Selenium," *Acres USA*, June 2007: 37(6), 38-44.

Josephson, Ramona, "E gets an 'F,'" *Chatelaine*, June 2006: 290.

Juhn, Mark S., "Oral Creatine Supplementation and Athletic Performance: A Critical Review," *Clinical Journal of Sports Medicine*, 1998: 8(4), 286-297.

Kang, J.H., N. Cook, et al, "A Randomized Trial of Vitamin E Supplementation and Cognitive Function in Women," *Archives of Internal Medicine*, 2006: 166, 2462-2468.

Kijkhuizen, Marjoleine A., Frank T Wieringa, et al, "Zinc Plus B-carotene Supplementation of Pregnant Women Is Superior to B-carotene Alone in Improving Vitamin A Status in Both Mothers and Infants," *American Journal of Clinical Nutrition*, Nov. 2004, 80(5),1299-1307.

Kim, Young-In, "Folic Acid Fortification and Supplementation—Good for Some but Not So Good for Others," *Nutrition Reviews*, Nov. 2007: 65(11), 504-511.

Klotter, Jule "Epigenetics," *Townsend Letter*, Feb./Mar. 2007: 28.

Klotter, Jule, "Selenium Supplements & Keep Hope Alive," *Townsend Letter*, May 2004: 250:23, citing Mark Konlee, *Journal of Immunity*, Spring 2003.

Kris-Etherton, P.M., A.H. Lichtenstein, et al, "Antioxidant Vitamin Supplements and Cardiovascular Disease," *Circulation*, 2004: 110, 637-641.

Lawlor, Debbie A., George Davey Smith, et al, "Those Confounded Vitamins: What Can We Learn from the Differences Between Observational Versus Randomized Trial Evidence?," *The Lancet*, 22 May 2004: 363(9422), 1724-1727.

"L-carnitine and Coenzyme Q10," *Alternative Medicine Alert*, Nov. 2001: 4(11), S1-S2.

Lee, Duk-Hee, Aaron R Folsom, et al, "Does Supplemental Vitamin C Increase Cardiovascular Disease Risk in Women with Diabetes?," *American Journal of Clinical Nutrition*, Nov. 2004: 80(5), 1194-1200.

Levin, Buck, "Antioxidants: Redefining Their Roles," *Integrative Medicine*, Dec. 2006/ Jan. 2007: 5(6), 28.

Li, Jialiang, Kirsten L. Molldrem, et al, "Lutein and B-carotene from Lutein-containing Yellow Carrots are Bioavailable in Humans," *American Journal of Clinical Nutrition*, July 2004: 80(1),131-136.

Li, Yi, and Herb E. Schellhorn, "New Developments and Novel Therapeutic Perspectives for Vitamin C," *The Journal of Nutrition*, Oct. 2007: 137(10), 2171-2184.

Liebman, Bonnie "Confusion at the Vitamin Counter," *Nutrition Action Health Letter*, Nov. 2007, 34(9), 1-6.

Lichtenstein, Alice H., and Robert M. Russell, "Essential Nutrients: Food or Supplements?", *Journal of the American Medical Association*, 20 July 2005: 294(3), 351-358.

Lorenzen, Janne K., Christian Molgaard, et al, "Calcium Supplementation for 1 y Does Not Reduce Body Weight or Fat Mass in Young Girls," *American Journal of Clinical Nutrition*, Jan. 2006: 83(1), 18-23.

Lyons, Graham H., James C.R. Stangoulis, et al, "Exploiting Micronutrient Interaction To Optimize Biofortification Programs: The Case for Inclusion of Selenium and Iodine in the *HarvestPlus* Program," *Nutrition Reviews*, June 2004: 62(6), 247-252.

Maseregian, Nancy Nairi, et al, *International Journal of Cancer*, Mar. 2007, cited by *Tufts University Health & Nutrition Letter*, June 2007: 25(4), 6.

Mason, Joel, "Researchers Weigh Benefits, Risks of Grain Fortification," *Nutrition Week*, 23 July 2007, 37(4), 6-7.

Massey, Linda, "Safety of Vitamin C," *American Journal of Clinical Nutrition*, Aug. 2005: 82(2), 488.

Massey, Linda K., Michael Liebman, et al, "Ascorbate Increases Human Oxaluria and Kidney Stone Risk," *Journal of Nutrition*, July 2005: 135(7), 1673-1677.

Masterjohn, Chris, "From Seafood to Sunshine," *Wise Traditions*, Fall 2006: 7(3), 14-33.

McKay, Diane, "Vitamin E Supplementation: An Update," *Alternative Medicine Alert*, Apr. 2007: 10(4), 37-42.

Mickleborough, Timothy D., Interview by Kirk Hamilton, VitaSearch.com, Mar. 2008.

"Missing from the Evidence for Antioxidants and Heart Health: Evidence," *Tufts University Health & Nutrition Letter*, Oct. 2004: 22(8), 2.

Moreno-Reyes, Rodrigo, Dominique Egrise, et al, "Iodine Deficiency Mitigates Growth Retardation and Osteopenia in Selenium-deficient Rats," *Journal of Nutrition*, Mar. 2006: 136(3), 595-600.

Morris, Martha Savaria, Paul F. Jacques, et al, "Cognitive Impairment in Older Americans in the Age of Folic Acid Fortification," *American Journal of Clinical Nutrition*, July 2007: 86(1), 265-269.

"Multis for Men: More Is Not Better," *Environmental Nutrition*, Aug. 2007: 30(8):3.

Nick, Gina L., "Impact of Glutamine-rich Foods on Immune Function," *Townsend Letter*, Apr. 2002: 225, 148-154.

"NIH Expert Panel Says Jury's Still out on Multivitamins," *Tufts University Health & Nutrition Letter*, Aug: 2006: 24(6):1-2.

Nishimuta, Mamoru, Naoko Kodama, et al, "Balance of Magnesium Positively Correlates with That of Calcium," *Journal of the American College of Nutrition*, Dec. 2004: 23(6), 768S-770S.

"Ask the Experts: Should I Take a Magnesium Supplement?," *UC Berkeley Wellness Letter*, " Jan. 2007: 23(4), 7.

"No Days Off," *Consumer Magazines Digest*, Feb. 2008: 20(2), 7.

"Not Much Evidence for Taking Multivitamins and, in Some Cases, Studies Show Harm," *Health Facts,* July 2006: 31(7):5-6.

"Nutrition from the Kitchen, not the Lab," *Tufts University Health & Nutrition Letter,* Nov. 2005: 23(9), 1-2.

Parker, Robert S., Letter to the editor, *Nutrition Reviews,* Mar. 2007: 65(3), 139.

Parsons, Greg, "The Importance of Mineral Supplements," *Acres USA,* Sept. 2003: 33(9), 30-31.

Pfeiffer, Christine M., Clifford L. Johnson, et al, "Trends in Blood Folate and Vitamin B$_{12}$ Concentrations in the United States, 1988-2004," *American Journal of Clinical Nutrition,* Sept. 2007: 86(3), 718-727.

Penniston, K.L., and S.A. Tanumihardjo, "Vitamin A in Dietary Supplements and Fortified Foods: Too Much of a Good Thing?," *Journal of the American Dietetic Association,* Sept. 2003: 103(9),1185-1187.

"Phenylalanine and Lysine," *Alternative Medicine Alert,* Jan. 2002: 5(1), S1-S2.

"Potassium: Making it Add Up," *UC Berkeley Wellness Letter,* Aug. 2004: 20(11), 3.

Quinlivan, Eoin, P., and Jesse F. Gregory III, "Reassessing Folic Acid Consumption Patterns in the United States (1999-2004): Potential Effect on Neural Tube Defects and Overexposure to Folate," *The American Journal of Clinical Nutrition,* Dec. 2007: 86(6), 1773-1779.

Quinn, Linda J., "Getting the Parts from the Whole," *Eating Well,* Fall 2003: 2(2), 21-22.

Reed, Michael C., H. Frederik Nijhout, et al, "A Mathematical Model Gives Insights into Nutritional and Genetic Aspects of Folate-mediated One-carbon Metabolism," *Journal of Nutrition,* Oct. 2006: 136(10), 2653-2661.

Renwick, A.G., "Toxicology of Micronutrients: Adverse Effects and Uncertainty," *The Journal of Nutrition,* Feb. 2006: supplement, 136(2S-I), 493S-501S.

Rogers, Sherry A., "The Folate Fiasco," *Total Wellness,* June 2007: 5-6.

Rogers, Sherry A., "Infections in Summer?," *Total Wellness,* Aug. 2007: 4.

Roughead, Aamzam K., Carol A Zito, et al, "Inhibitory Effects of Dietary Calcium on the Initial Uptake and Subsequent Retention of Heme and Nonheme Iron in Humans: Comparisons Using an Intestinal Lavage Method," *American Journal of Clinical Nutrition,* Sept. 2005: 82(3), 589-597.

Rowen, Robert Jay, "Vitamin E's Rediscovered Twin Unclogs Arteries and Lowers Cholesterol," *Second Opinion,* Dec. 2007: 17(12), 1-5.

Samuel, Neena, "The Vitamin Myth," *Reader's Digest,* Nov. 2007: 85.

Schardt, David, "Potassium: Bones, Stones, & Strokes on the Line," *Nutrition Action Health Letter,* Dec. 2004: 31(10), 8-9.

Schernhammer, Eva, et al, *Cancer Research,* 2007: 67(11), 5553-5560.

Schulman, Steven P., Lewis C. Becker, et al, "L-arginine Therapy in Acute Myocardial Infarction," *Journal of the American Medical Association,* 4 Jan. 2006: 295(1), 58-64.

Shin, Laura, "Minerals 101," *Natural Health,* Mar. 2006: 36(3), 93-96.

Smith, David, "Folic Acid Fortification: the Good, the Bad, and the Puzzle of Vitamin B$_{12}$," *American Journal of Clinical Nutrition,* Jan. 2007: 85(1), 3-5.

Smith, David, Young-In Kim, and Helga Refsum, "Is Folic Acid Good For Everyone?," *American Journal of Clinical Nutrition*, Mar. 2008: 87(3), 517-33.

Smith, Julie, Marianne Empson, et al, "Recurrent Anaphylaxis to Synthetic Folic Acid," *Lancet*, 25 Aug. 2007: 370(9588), 652.

"Stay Nimble with C," *Natural Health*, Oct. 2004: 34(10), 22.

Stechmiller, J.K., B. Childress, et al, "Arginine Immunonutrition in Critically Ill Patients: A Clinical Dilemma," *American Journal of Critical Care*, Jan. 2004: 13(1), 17-23.

Stolzenberg-Soloman, Rachael, Shih-Chem Chang, et al, "Folate Intake, Alcohol Use, and Postmenopausal Breast Cancer Risk," *American Journal of Clinical Nutrition*, Apr. 2006: 83(4), 895-904.

Stranges, S., et al, "Effects of Long-term Selenium Supplementation, the Incidence of Type 2 Diabetes, *Annals of Internal Medicine*, 2007: 147, 217-223.

Sullivan, Jerome L., "Long-term Risks of Increased Use of Intravenous Iron," *The Lancet*, 11 Aug. 2007: 370(9586), 481-482.

Talegawkar, Sameera A., Elizabeth J. Johnson, et al, "Total *A*-tocopherol Intakes Are Associated with Serum *A*-tocopherol Concentrations," *Journal of Nutrition*, Oct. 2007: 137(10), 2297-2303.

"The Antioxidant Controversy," *Duke Medicine HealthNews*, May 2007: 13(5), 1, 11.

"The Power of Blueberries and… ," *HealthNews*, Oct. 2004: 10(10), 8-9.

Townsend Letter, Aug./Sept. 2006: 277/278:51-52.

Traver, Maret G., "How Much Vitamin E?...Just Enough!," *American Journal of Clinical Nutrition*, Nov. 2006: 84(5), 959-960.

Troen, Aron M., Breeana Mitchell, et al, "Unmetabolized Folic Acid in Plasma Is Associated with Reduced Natural Killer Cell Cytotoxicity Among Postmenopausal Women," *Journal of Nutrition*, Jan. 2006: 136(1), 189-194.

"Tryptophan," *Alternative Medicine Alert*, Dec. 2001: 4(12), S1-S2.

Ulrich, Cornelia M., and John D. Potter, "Folate and Cancer—Timing Is Everything," *Journal of the American Medical Association*, 6 June 2007: 297(21), 2408-2409.

"Unsung Form of Vitamin E Proving to Be Important to Your Health," *Environmental Nutrition*, Nov. 2006: 29(11), 7.

"Vitamin A: 'Magic Bullet' That Can Backfire," *Tufts University Health & Nutrition Letter*, Feb. 2005: 22(2):4-5;

"Vitamin C May Help Prevent Arthritis," *Health News*, Nov. 2004: 10(11), 7.

"Vitamins for the Brain," *Consumer Magazine Digest*, Oct. 2007: 19(10), 6.

Wald, D.S., J.K. Morris, et al, "Folic Acid, Homocysteine, and Cardiovascular Disease: Judging Causality in the Face of Inconclusive Trial Evidence," *British Medical Journal*, 2006: 333, 1114-1117.

Wannamethee, S. Goya, Fordon D.O. Lower, et al, "Associations of Vitamin C Status, Fruit and Vegetable Intakes, and Markers of Inflammation and Hemostasis," *American Journal of Clinical Nutrition*, Mar. 2006: 83,(3), 657-674.

Wasantwisut, Emorn, Pattanee Winichagoon, et al, "Iron and Zinc Supplementation Improved Iron and Zinc Status, but Not Physical Growth, of Apparently Healthy, Breast-fed Infants in Rural Communities of Northeast Thailand," *Journal of Nutrition*, Sept. 2006: 136(9), 2405-2411.

"Wellness Facts," *UC Berkeley Wellness Letter*, Dec. 2007: 24(3), 1.

Wenzel, K-G, and RJ Pataracchia, *The Earth's Gift to Medicine*, Alton, Ontario. KOS Publishing, Inc, 2005.

"What's New About Zinc," *UC Berkeley Wellness Letter*, Apr. 2004: 20(7), 7.

Wieringa, F.T., J. Berger, et al, "Combined Iron and Zinc Supplementation in Infants Improved Iron and Zinc Status, but Interactions Reduced Efficacy in a Multicountry Trial in Southeast Asia," *Journal of Nutrition*, 2007: 137(2), 466-471.

Wolfe, Sydney M., "Do Not Use Amino Acid Dietary Supplement L-arginine After a Heart Attack," *Worst Pills, Best Pills News*, Apr. 2006: 12(4), 27-29.

Wright, Jonathan V., "Taking B_{12}? Don't Forget the Methylfolate!," *Nutrition & Healing*, Sept. 2007. 14(7): 3.

Wright, Margaret E., Karla A. Lawson, et al, "Higher Baseline Serum Concentrations of Vitamin E Are Associated with Lower Total and Cause-specific Mortality in the Alpha-Tocopherol, Beta-Carotene Cancer Prevention Study," *American Journal of Clinical Nutrition*, Nov. 2006: 84(5), 1200-1207.

Wysong, Randy, "A New and Potent Sun Vitamin Supplement," *Townsend Letter*, Feb./Mar. 2006: 271/272, 73-76.

Ziaei, Saedeh, et al, *International Journal of Obstetrics and Gynaecology*, 2007: 114(6), 684-688.

Zimmermann, Michael B., Ralf Biebinger, et al, "Vitamin A Supplementation in Children with Poor Vitamin A and Iron Status Increases Erythropoietin and Hemoglobin Concentrations Without Changing Total Body Iron," *American Journal of Clinical Nutrition*, Sept. 2006: 84(3), 580-586.

"Zinc Can Help You Think," *Health*, Sept. 2005: 19(7), 37.

YOU CAN SEE THE DIFFERENCE

The pictures on the followng pages are called *chromatograms*. The process to make them records, on specially made filter papers, a stain made visible by a reagent (a substance used to detect the presence of another substance) The chromatograms reveal distinct differences in colors, rings, spikes, and other patterns that relate to the qualitative and biological values of a substance. These chromatograms illustrate differences between soils, foods, and nutrients. They show how Nature's products are so much more beautiful and complex, containing biological activity, harmony, and synergy. Human products cannot come close to Nature's work and are clearly lacking in many important areas.

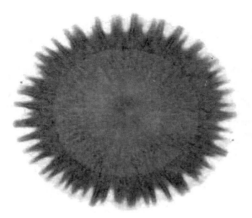 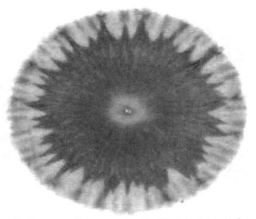

1a. Chemically-treated soil

1b. Organically-treated soil. Rich in microlife, humus, and organic matter.

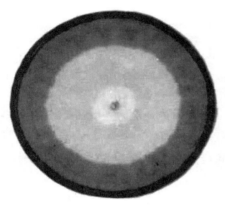 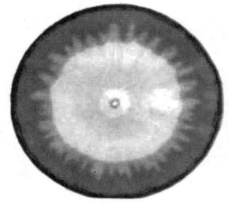

2a. Young green leaf from a corn stalk grown on chemically-treated soil. Faded pattern of middle ring indicates lower enzyme activity.

2b. Young green leaf from a corn stalk grown on organically-treated soil. The jagged inner edge of the middle ring shows enzyme & biological activity.

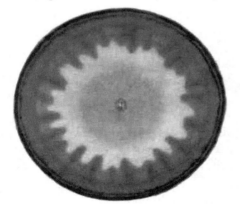 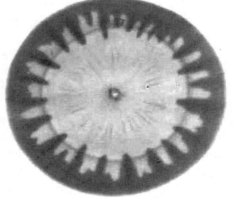

3a. Young green leaves of oat plants grown on chemically-treated soil. Lower protein and enzyme activity.

3b. Young green leaves of oat plants grown on organically-treated soil. Stronger protein and enzyme activity.

138

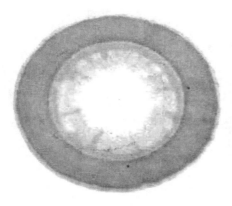

4a. Refined "white" sugar (sucrose). Missing all intrinsic factors present in raw unrefined sugar.

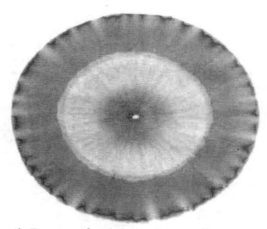

4b. Raw, unrefined "brown" sugar. Contains intrinsic factors and enzymes.

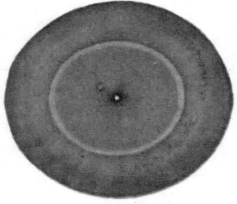

5a. Chemically-refined sugar (dextrose). Lacks nutritional value.

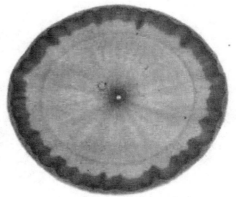

5b. Old-fashioned molasses. More nutrients indicated by wider, more wavy outer zone and slight radiating inner area.

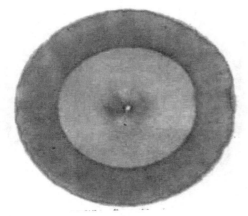

6a. Bleached refined "white" flour. Lacks nutrient and enzyme formations. Little remains of original quality of whole wheat seeds.

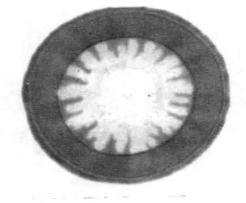

6b. Whole unbleached wheat flour, organically grown. Contains natural components, nutrients, and enzymes.

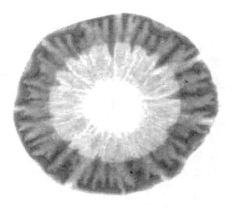

7a. Pasteurized whole milk. Paler, missing some natural nutritional factors.

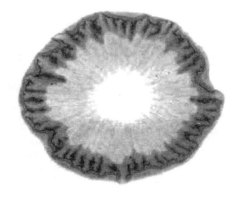

7b. Raw whole milk. Plenty of proteins, vitamins, minerals, and other nutrients.

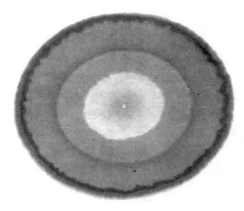

8a. A popular soft drink. Outer edge shows the sugar. Not much else inside.

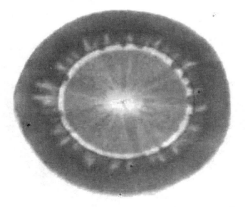

8b. Fresh organic orange juice. Presence of enzymes, vitamin C complex, and other natural constituents.

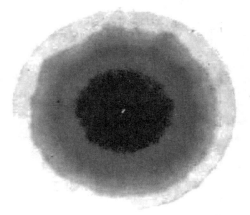

9a. Margarine. Lacks nutrient and enzyme formation.

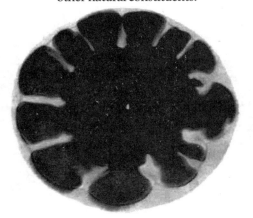

9b. Butter, fresh from unpasteurized milk. Patterns and colors indicate many natural factors and nutrient influences.

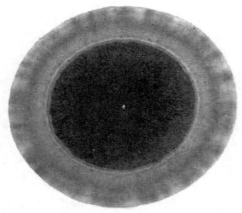

10a. Ascorbic acid (so-called "vitamin C"). No biologically active ingredients.

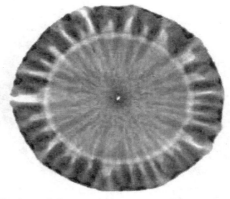

10b. Acerola berry, rich in vitamin C complex, containing synergistic nutrients and enzyme activity.

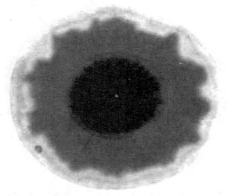

11a. D-alpha tocopherol, a small part of the vitamin E complex. Intrinsic factors are missing because it is refined, only a fraction of the real whole complex.

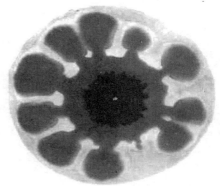

11b. Wheat germ oil, unheated—a natural source of vitamin E complex. Contains all tocopherols, tocotrienols, fatty acids, enzymes, and other intrinsic factors. Note similarity to butter.

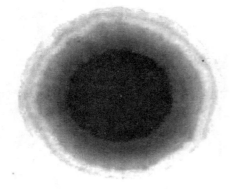

12a. Synthetic vitamin A made from refined, chemically-altered lemon grass root. It is missing the winged or leaf pattern that shows up in natural oils.

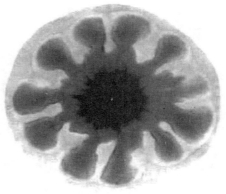

12b. Cod liver oil, unrefined. See the winged or leaf pattern found in all natural oils and fats. Excellent source of vitamins A and D as well as omega-3 fats.

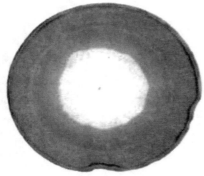

13a. Vitamin B complex, synthetic mixture of manufactured B vitamin parts. No spikes to indicate enzyme formations or biologically-active natural factors.

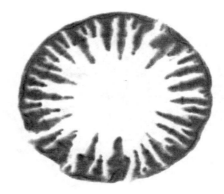

13b. Natural, food-source vitamin B complex. Long jagged "teeth" indicate natural nutritional factors, good protein, and strong enzyme activity.

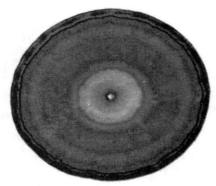

14a. Mixture of synthetic vitamins and inorganic (not food source) minerals. Totally lacking in biologically-active natural factors and enzyme formations.

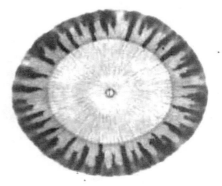

14b. Juice from young green barley, wheat, oat, and rye grasses. Center radiation and jagged spikes show excellent biological activity, nutrients, and enzymes.

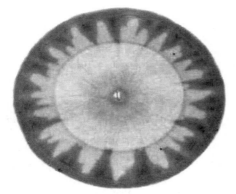

15a. A so-called "natural" dietary supplement containing synthetic vitamins and inorganic minerals. Indications of enzyme interference and lack of food function.

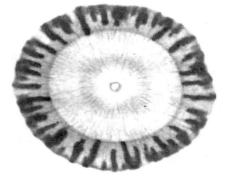

15b. A real food supplement of vegetable juices, bone meal, yeast, and fish oil. Evidence of enzyme function and presence of natural factors found in real foods.

Chapter Nine

WHY TAKE SUPPLEMENTS?

Suppose you decide, beginning today, to eat only healthful real foods? Do you still need to take supplements? Ideally, you shouldn't need to take any dietary supplements *if* the following conditions are true for you:

- if you have been eating nutrient-dense, organic whole foods most or all of your life,
- if your mother ate the best foods and got all the nutrients she needed for herself and for you while she was pregnant,
- if your parents were extremely healthy,
- if you had frequently been outdoors in sunshine and clean, fresh air,
- if you lived and worked in places where there were few, if any, toxins,
- if you never used tobacco or drank large amounts of alcohol,
- if you didn't experience illness or didn't develop any health conditions or diseases,
- if you never took drugs frequently or for long periods,
- if you did not endure large amounts of stress in your life...

Well, if you had this healthy, ideal lifestyle and diet plus you picked good parents with excellent genetic disposition, then you wouldn't need supplements. If you're typical of most people living in this industrialized age, exposed to all the common pollutants and toxins, eating a standard American diet (SAD), and living a lifestyle full of stress, then it's likely you need to take some real food supplements. This is because you probably have deficiencies or imbalances and need some extra help to 'catch up' on what you don't have enough of and which your body requires. If you can improve your diet and nutrient intake, develop a healthy lifestyle, reduce stress, and avoid many toxins, then you could no doubt stop taking supplements eventually.

In the chapter, "What Happened To Our Food?", some of the atrocities of agriculture and food processing were mentioned. All of these things—from industrialized farming to refining and chemical adulteration of our food—impoverish nutrients that should be or were in the foods and impoverish our bodies of vital health-giving nourishment.

Additionally, "fresh" foods are stored, sometimes for long periods of time. "Fresh" in your grocery store does not mean the item was just harvested, but that it will spoil before frozen or cooked items do. Then we take our stored items home and store them some more. An orange sitting in your refrigerator can lose up to 60% of its vitamin C content in a few days. Canned, pre-cooked, and other prepared foods have been heated and packaged so they will stay on the shelves long enough for you to pluck them off. But the heavy-duty cooking drains nutrients. Then you take such a prepared food home and cook it again.

Depending on our age, you and I are among the members of the first or second generation living on this earth that has spent every single day exposed to some poisons and/or toxins. Harmful chemicals can be found in your body and in my body—to various degrees, of course. We can limit our exposure, but we can't totally avoid it. Toxic chemicals are all around us now, from agricultural chemicals to building materials, from household items to industrial pollutants.

Most people these days spend most of their time indoors in artificial light, often in front of a television or computer which emits another artificial light. Not only do we miss out on the fresh air and connection to nature, but we also miss out on the benefits of natural sunlight. I think of sunlight as a vital part of a healthy lifestyle. People with wintertime blues, anxiety, or hyperactivity can benefit from spending time out in the sunshine. And sunlight is our best source of vitamin D which our skin and bodies make from the natural light. Without enough vitamin D our bones suffer and we may become more susceptible to muscle aches and weakness, balance problems, heart disease, certain cancers (like breast and prostate), as well as numerous other health problems. Lack of sunlight even influences levels of some hormones.

Then there are drugs. Not only do enormous amounts of excreted and disposed drugs get into the environment (where they are having powerfully negative impacts in ecosystems), but they have negative effects on our bodies that use up nutrients. About 1,000 prescription drugs and many over-the-counter drugs are *known* to deplete one or more nutrients in humans. They include blood pressure medications, birth control pills, estrogen replacements, ulcer drugs, anti-convulsants, cholesterol-lowering statins, beta blockers, antibiotics, anti-inflammatory drugs, some anti-depressants, and many more. For example, birth control pills and estrogen replacements deplete several B vitamins, vitamin C, zinc, magnesium, and more. Anti-inflammatory steroid drugs decrease magnesium, potassium, zinc, copper, selenium, and possibly vitamins C and D. Statins are well known to significantly decrease coenzyme Q-10, a deficiency of which can contribute to heart disease. Blood pressure medications can deplete vitamin B_6, sodium, potassium and other nutrients; diuretics deplete potassium, magnesium, calcium, zinc, B6, B1, other B vitamins, and vitamin C. Antibiotics have been shown to adversely affect levels of numerous vitamins and minerals.

- Percentage of Americans who take dietary supplements: 73

- Percentage of them who experienced an adverse reaction they believed might be related to supplements use::   4

> (mostly high-potency, synthetic, contaminated, adulterated, or caused allergic reaction)

Passage of the Dietary Supplement and Health Education Act (DSHEA) in 1994 stimulated growth of the supplement industry.

- Number of supplement products on the market in 1994:   about 4,000
- Number of supplement products on the market in 1999: about 29,000

> (a current figure is not available)

- Sales of dietary supplements in 1994: $4 billion
- Sales of dietary supplements in 2006: $21 billion
- In contrast, annual sales of pharmaceuticals (drugs): $200 billion

("Regulating vitamins and herbs," *Health Facts*, Oct. 2007, Vol.32, No.10:5. Saldanha, Leila G. "The Dietary Supplement Marketplace," *Nutrition Today*, Mar./Apr. 2007, 42(2):52-53)

Number of people in the US who died as a result of taking a prescription drug in 2005:   5,107
Number of people who suffered a serious adverse reaction resulting in disability, hospital care, or birth defect during 2005:   89, 842

(These figures represent a 2.7 times increase in only eight years. The Food and Drug Administration received reports of a total of 467,809 deaths and serious adverse reactions between 1998 and 2005. *Archives of Internal Medicine*, 2007, 167:1752-59.)

All drugs are toxic; many are poisons. It's just that we take doses small enough so they don't kill us. And the vast majority of drugs don't heal diseases; rather, they control symptoms by introducing chemical mediators, at certain levels, into the body. Nearly all pharmaceuticals are not a normal part of the diet, not a food by any stretch of the imagination. They take, rather than give nutrition. Don't get me wrong. There are times when drugs can save a life or alleviate suffering. But drugs are overused, unnecessarily used, and used more for convenience instead of putting forth the time and effort to build true health and wellness.

One of my Dad's neighbors, an elderly lady, asked my Dad (who is 90 years old) if he takes any drugs. He told her he did not. Stunned, she asked, "What do you do?" He explained that he ate good wholesome foods and took some real food supplements. She frowned and spurted out that she couldn't be bothered. She'd rather take drugs. From what my Dad knows, she takes about nine different prescribed medications, some of which were probably prescribed to mask side effects of others. I won't list all her health problems here, though I know several are quite serious. But I was a little disheartened by her lack of willingness to do something more positive about her health.

Your needs for nutrients skyrocket if you have an illness, especially a long-standing health condition like diabetes, cancer, cardiovascular disease, arthritis, inflammatory digestive disease, asthma, or others. Even the common cold can greatly increase your need for many nutrients for a while. Pregnancy and nursing certainly require an abundance of nutritional goodies.

Bottom line: There is an awful lot of evidence that "suggests" that most Americans are deficient in various nutrients. This is particularly true when there is a health issue. Numerous scientific studies have already shown this.

It makes me very sad and angry that the supplement industry (including companies that produce herbal supplements) is bent towards making drugs out of supplements. The same is true of the food industry which has introduced products classified as "nutraceuticals," a word that attempts to combine *nutri*tion with pharma*ceuticals* (drugs). People may want natural remedies. But, far too often, what they are getting are chemicals manufactured in some laboratory or chemicals isolated from an herb or food, which are then sometimes laced with a sprinkling of food or herb powder. The synthetic or separated chemicals are not real whole food packages. They behave much more like drugs in the body.

Okay, so sometimes a separate nutrient may be required if there is a dire need. For instance, someone with severe iron-deficiency anemia needs a bunch of iron for a while, to catch up. But such a person also needs real food sources of iron along with other nutrients and other substances that help with the absorption of and proper use of the iron in the body. And, after a period of time, use of any separate iron should be discontinued while the real food sources should be continued. Otherwise, imbalances and biochemical glitches may occur.

Many of you folks are seeking some supplements that will protect you from disease, help treat a condition or illness that you have, prolong your life or prevent signs of aging. But human-made chemicals won't do that. The best thing is to consume the fresh foods and herbs that can give our bodies all the authentic natural materials needed to proceed with healing, with repair, with detoxification, with maintenance or preservation. Real foods are *not* nutraceuticals.

"Nutraceutical" refers to any substance originally "found" within real foods that can be ground up, extracted, concentrated, imitated, and otherwise stuffed into easy-to-swallow pills or added to foods. That brings us to "functional foods" (or "pharmafoods"), synonymous with nutraceuticals. These are foods containing added compounds with supposed health benefits. They can be "fortified" with or are promoted as:

 * Vitamins, minerals and other separated, synthetic or inorganic materials like folic acid in your bread, calcium added to your orange juice, added fiber (sometimes wood cellulose) in cereal.

 * Plant stenols or sterol esters to reduce cholesterol such as Benecol spreads.

 * Beneficial bacteria such as added cultures in yogurt.

 * Herbs or separate chemicals extracted from herbs like ginseng or echinacea found in juices, teas, and bottled waters.

 * Magic foods such as energy drinks with white tea, energy bars made mostly of refined sugars.

 * Nutrients or pharmaceutical medicines (theoretically) produced by genetic engineering (unnatural tampering with Nature).

 * Innumerable other newly thought-of or newly developed magic elixirs.

Marion Nestle, PhD, professor of nutrition at New York University, says, "Functional foods tend to promise miracles, but I see them as about marketing, not health." Many other nutrition scientists and many of us practicing nutritionists down here in the trenches are, shall we say, just as skeptical. There are lots of false claims, and there are lots of marketing ploys (products claiming to be 'calming' or 'relaxing', for example, when it's difficult to say what's really going on). But these marketing tactics work. People are buying it.

"Functional foods" aren't new; just the name is. Iodized salt, for instance, has been around since the 1920s. Wheaties have been "the breakfast of champions" for years because of the synthetic chemical "nutrients" added. But with advancing technology, new types of ingredient manipulations are becoming possible. Diet Coke Plus is "fortified" with B vitamins, zinc and magnesium. Not only are the amounts tiny, but they are not whole food packages. HeartBar, a soy-based candy bar contains arginine and other additives. Glaceau Vitaminwater is enhanced with synthetic vitamins. Snapple tea is spiked with kava kava. Mars' CocoaVia chocolate bars contain calcium, folic acid, and other imitation vitamins.

Are we supposed to get all our nutrients from soda and cookies? I don't consider the additions as real food nutrients, and neither does your body. There is always the possibility of unexpected side effects too. You're much better off eating whole foods that naturally contain entire, complex nutrient packages that have a plethora of benefits rather than eating some mangled, manipulated, highly refined nonfood that has one or several added ingredients, even if they are herbs. Go for real foods.

Chocolate is getting some promotional press as a "health food." Are chocolate kisses and truffles really treatments for cardiovascular wellbeing—yummy tasting solutions?

Chocolate manufacturers would like you to think so and they have financed some of the studies. While legitimate studies have indicated that dark chocolate, rich in flavanols improve the function of blood vessels, for instance, most chocolate you buy won't have this good stuff. Milk and white chocolate are often devoid of flavanols and offer no health benefits. Dark chocolate can be deceptive; manufacturers can darken the natural cocoa solids and remove the flavanols, which are bitter. Thus, dark-looking chocolate may have no flavanols. Even if flavanols are present, what about all the refined sugar that must be added to make the chocolate sweet enough? Refined sugars have been shown to be contributors to heart disease, overweight, and other banes. Don't be deceived by this any other processed-food promotions. Carrying home a cart-load of chocolate or any other processed food is not going to make you healthy no matter how tantalizing it seems.

If you take isolated (unaccompanied by its natural food companions) or synthetic (fabricated by humans rather than by Nature) so-called nutrients or buy into the nutraceutical, functional food ploys, you are being fooled. You may feel a rush of energy, for example. When people contact me and tell me they "found" a supplement that gave them a boost within a couple of days—"isn't this wonderful?"—I cringe. Real nutrition doesn't work like that. Real nutrition takes time. Nature is slow. I'm sorry, but that's the way it works. And Nature knows what it's doing. When you give your body real nutrients as whole natural food packages, you are supplying fuel or nourishment for your cells. The cells gradually improve their function, the tissues gradually become healthier, and you gradually feel better. It may be several weeks or a couple of months before you begin to experience the improvements. With the level of deficiencies that we are dealing with these days, it often takes many months or even a year or two before a person can totally overcome them.

Unfortunately, we have been programmed into a drug mentality. Fast acting. Quick relief. We want the same thing from supplements. Yeah, you can get it from some supplements, but they aren't real food supplements. They aren't going to really and truly nourish those cells of yours the way they need to be nourished. What you are going to do is give them a broken part or, worse still, an imitation part. The response of your body is much more like its response to a drug.

The rush to excrete as much of the nonfood (which may be interpreted by your body as toxic) substance from itself can give you a "high" that makes you feel energized for a little while. Whatever is left over has to be combined with real nutrients from your body to try to make something that resembles nourishment—using up nutrients that you can't afford to use up or lose. And/or there is the drug-like action. These chemical supplements may stimulate or suppress processes in the body, they may mask symptoms. But they can't produce the healing that real foods provide.

Real foods can be concentrated into real food supplements. Since we probably have not eaten the best, nutrient-dense, really fresh and clean real foods all our lives, and since we may have health issues that we want to deal with, then taking real food supplements may be helpful, at least for a while.

Picture this: You have been given the serious responsibility of filling a big vessel with thousands of materials that it needs to function properly. But, you goof off and don't do much. And you start throwing things in that don't belong. After a while, you notice some squeaks and clicks coming from the vessel. You look in and are shocked to see how low the level of needed materials is. So you panic and start heaving in anything you find in the area that you think is similar to the materials you were supposed to be putting in all along. Now there are clangs and crashes. You finally realize that you need to get back to putting in the materials that were really needed all along. You begin to put in these materials, but you can't catch up to the amounts required because of all the time you neglected doing your job properly. You need extra help.

Of course, the vessel is your body. The extra help you may need are real food supplements—in addition to the essential foundation of a good diet of wholesome real foods. Look at the label of the supplement. Does it contain things like "carrots, broccoli, kale, liver, kelp, beets," and other words you know that identify foods? Be careful when you read the label of an herbal supplement. If the word "standardized" is used, it may mean that a chemical separated from an herb (thought to be the "active ingredient") is added to the batch used to make the supplement. This can create imbalances as well as lessen the actual amount of whole herb you get. "Standardized" can also mean a method of processing that assures you that you are getting all the ingredients in a biologically active form and sufficient concentration. Know your source.

Buyer Beware:

The words "all natural" on a label don't mean a darn thing. I have often told clients that my desk is all natural, but I wouldn't want to eat it. And labels on supplements can read "all natural" even when they contain ingredients that are entirely synthetic, made in a laboratory.

There are some supplements on the market that promote the idea that they are food concentrates, but, in reality, they aren't. For example, some labels read: "in a food base." That usually means it contains separated nutrients (often chemical imitations manufactured in laboratories, not made by Nature) combined with a paltry bit of food. They are not much different than the plain isolated, synthetic types. Adding insult to injury, sometimes the "food base" is barley grass or wheat grass, mere fillers. Cows and goats can digest grass. We humans can't digest grass. We can use barley or wheat grass *juice*, but not the whole grass. The whole grass is cheap to put in supplements, though it can boost the price you pay.

A few supplement companies have come up with a method of making supplements that really sounds good...until you look deeper. The products are promoted as whole food supplements. They say this because manufactured mock vitamins and/or inorganic (non-food) minerals are incorporated into growing, living yeasts. They begin with a "soup" of

149

"USP nutrients"—the chemical imitation or non-food types—along with some whole food concentrates, water, soy or a grain. Yeast is put in to begin fermenting the soup. Plant enzymes are added to break the cell walls of the yeast. At the end of the process, the "USP nutrients" are said to be completely "biotransformed into dynamic whole food complexes." The claim is that "probiotic organisms" like bacteria and yeasts can "give life" to dead, inert chemical USP nutrients. Why does a vision of Frankenstein come into my head?

Yes, I have some trouble with these claims. First of all, I look at the labels and see various nutrients listed (depending on the particular product) in amounts that would not be contained in one tablet of a real food concentrate. For instance, vitamin C at 60 milligrams, vitamin D at 400 IU, niacin at 20 milligrams, iron at 5 milligrams and so on. These amounts are too large for foods that could be pressed into a tablet or poured into a capsule. When there are 25 or so "nutrients" listed in such amounts for one tablet, I have to conclude that they are *not* what would naturally occur in real foods. Rather, they are the very same "USP nutrients" put in the yeast-fed soup. They haven't changed except that they may be absorbed into the body easier because of the process they have been put through. They are still separate or imitation chemicals, not natural complexes. They are still missing all the naturally-occurring synergists of food that the yeast, soy, or other ingredients in the "soup" cannot give them because they are not truly a part of food. They remain broken chemicals. The synergy of whole foods was never in them. Putting them into yeast doesn't change that. You can't make a real, whole food from manufactured chemicals. Living things can only be produced from living things.

Yes, the yeast may incorporate chemical "nutrients" into itself. But does that really change the chemical into a food? That's like saying pesticides and herbicides applied to growing plants are "changed" into foods. The plants may absorb them, but the toxic chemicals don't morph into healthful food. Also, these supplements, being yeast-based, must be heated to "kill" the yeast (if you eat live yeast with other foods, you make beer in your belly). Heat destroys the enzymes, the catalysts that help nutrients "work." It also destroys water-soluble vitamins and some amino acids. Yeast itself is wonderfully nutritious. Putting some real food into a supplement is also wonderful. But don't think that chemicals added are miraculously metamorphized into whole foods. If the manufacturers put aspirin or cocaine into yeast, would these drugs be changed into foods? If you listed the milligrams of aspirin or cocaine on the label, would you assume that they are simply normal natural ingredients of yeast or another food? No way.

Ain't nothin' like the real thing. So we get back to natural, whole foods being the best source of real nutrition. Real nutrients appear in small amounts in real foods. They are extremely potent—powerful—due to their synergistic cooperation. They are interconnected, inter-related. If you break them apart, they lose their power, their function. Together, as a webwork, they provide food for your cells, food your body recognizes and uses as nourishment. So the best nutritional supplements are made of real foods. Period.

By the way, I think that one of the best real food supplements you can get is freshly-made juice. When you juice fresh vegetables and fruits, you obtain a concentrated amount of many nutrients. This valuable source of heavy-duty nutrition is very easily absorbed and assimilated. Often they prove to be invaluable for people with digestive difficulties or serious health conditions. Fresh juices also juice-up detoxification. And they support healing processes.

Some people have expressed concern that fresh juices contain too much "sugar" (referring to the natural sugars that appear in the veggies and fruits) because, without most of the fiber to slow down absorption of these sugars, they might disrupt blood sugar processing in the body. While some people may not be able to handle a large amount of fruit juice, most people do just fine with fresh juices, particularly if they combine vegetables and fruit. Numerous juices from around the world have been noted to have healthful, therapeutic properties. Many alternative-type clinics administer fresh juices to their patients with amazing results. The Gerson Institute Clinic, for example, is well known for their therapeutic program which has helped thousands of people over the span of many decades. People with cancer come to this clinic as well as folks with various other serious and chronic diseases. It is interesting that people with diabetes getting the Gerson Therapy have enjoyed vast improvements and even remission of their diabetes on this program. All patients are given freshly-made juices *thirteen times* a day. It doesn't appear that the juices mess up blood sugar metabolism.

Recent studies have indicated that juices are, indeed, therapeutic. Pomegranate juice has received positive press for preventing and aiding heart disease and cancer. Beetroot juice appears to lower blood pressure in those with hypertension. Cranberry juice (unsweetened) may actually reduce blood sugar in folks who experience blood sugar spikes after eating. A recent scientific study showed the health benefits of cherry juice, including the prevention of exercise-induced muscle damage. And it did not have any bad effects on blood sugar. Green leafy vegetables that are juiced provide oodles of nutrients—vitamins, minerals, phytochemicals, chlorophyll—that are good for every cell in your body. Carrots have been found to contain hundreds of beneficial nutrients. So drag out that juicer from the back of your kitchen cabinet. The preferred type of juicer is a "masticating" juicer. Juicers that perform with centrifugal force tend to oxidize the juice, so you don't get quite as many nutrients as you would from the masticating types. The best ones work slowly at between 70 and 90 RPM.

What should you juice? Get organic or at least locally grown produce. Carrots and apples for a start. Romaine and other kinds of lettuce (except iceberg), spinach, chard, kale, cabbage, small amounts of parsley, beetroot and beet greens (begin with small amounts of beetroot), dandelion greens, celery or whatever else is in season. In summer, you could add a bit of bell pepper, string beans, summer squash, or other vegetables, for example. Some adventurous types add a sliver of fresh ginger and/or garlic to liven up their drink. Others like to toss in a few leaves of their favorite fresh herb like cilantro, French sorrel, or lemon balm. I've even known a few who add lemon juice and a little lemon rind (if organic). Get creative. But be sure to include some green leafy vegetables. You can get 8 ounces a day or up to 32 ounces. Remember, you make juice as a supplement to, not a substitute for, fruits and vegetables in your diet.

Bottled juices are another story. "Supplements" of noni juice, goji berry juice, and mangosteen juice have been highly promoted of late. Although all such fruits are no doubt nutritious and good for you, once they are bottled, they lose a lot. Plus, they are promoted as "superfoods" and cure-alls. Sorry. They don't live up to the exorbitant claims. Other bottled juices (whether fruit or vegetable combos) are also not nearly as good as freshly made. They are almost always pasteurized, meaning they are heated to destroy all enzymes. Not only to you lose the wonderful enzymes that are important to the nutritional value, you lose many nutrients as well. Plus, the bottled versions become more and more acid-forming as they sit on the shelf. Freshly-made juices are very alkaline-forming in your body. We need more alkaline, less acid these days. You certainly don't have to worry about your fresh juice containing any additives or manufactured chemicals. Yes, making your own juice is a little time-consuming and requires a little planning, effort and clean-up. But you can't beat the benefits. Are you worth it? How about your children and family?

When you buy tablets or capsules or powered supplements, make sure to read the labels. For example: "Vitamin A acetate or palmitate" is not real vitamin A. "Beta-carotene" is not a carotene complex and may be synthetic. "Thiamine hydrochloride or mononitrate is not vitamin B_1. "Pyridoxine hydrochloride" is not vitamin B_6. "Niacin" is not vitamin B_3. "Asorbic acid" is not vitamin C complex. "Irradiated ergosterol" is not vitamin D. "Alpha or mixed tocopherols" are not vitamin E complex.

This list could continue. What you want to see is a list of real foods—words you understand. The amounts of certain nutrients may be required to be listed, but these amounts should be small. "50 milligrams" of each of the B vitamins is too high and uniform to be from foods, for instance. No food contains exactly 50 milligrams of each and every B vitamin. Single nutrients or nutrient "cocktails" are not the same as real food complexes. They are simply a tiny (often synthetic) part or groups of tiny parts in a form and in amounts that confuse rather than feed your body. They are not food.

The vast majority of supplements are made from isolated substances, such as sugar. If you see a label with a 2-part chemical name, like pyridoxine hydrochloride, calcium citrate, or magnesium oxide, it is usually a refined vitamin or mineral. The chemical structure of refined sugar (sucrose) is very similar to the chemical structure of ascorbic acid. Both are "simple" structures with many similarities. Ascorbic acid is made from corn syrup which is further refined and manipulated until it is about as far from natural as you can get. If you take supplements containing ascorbic acid or calcium ascorbate, you aren't getting food. You're getting a highly refined sugar. In a lab, you can convert sugar into ascorbic acid in only 4 basic steps. This is quite different from eating an orange. Even if a product claims to be a "whole food" supplement yet contains ascorbic acid as a source, you are not getting whole foods.

If you could see all the biochemical pathways in your body, you would be overwhelmed and mesmerized. If someone takes out, or puts in, one isolated nutrient in any one particular place in any of these pathways, it affects the entire system in some way. It's ecology—if you disturb one area, you affect the whole. So, studying the effects of single nutrients or combined nutrients and how they affect the body is not only not easy, but impossible. Taking single nutrients or nutrient cocktails is not only not wise, but disrupting.

For a true real food supplement, you want one that starts with high quality real foods. Then you want one in which the foods undergo only a minimal amount of processing, using low heat and maintaining the essential nature of the food components rather than high heat and processing that denatures (changes the structure or essence of) the original food. Real food supplements will not produce an immediate "bang." They won't give you a quick burst of energy, they won't put you to sleep, they won't instantaneously mask a symptom or cure a problem. They do not behave as drugs. Rather, they feed your cells so that your body can gradually repair, detoxify, balance, and heal. You will notice improvements by degrees, bit by bit, like climbing stairs. You will sense that you are becoming truly well.

Most of all, make sure you eat a nutritionally-rich diet of fresh, natural whole foods. Don't think that any supplement can replace real organically-raised food. It is your foundation for health. Honest-to-goodness food is much more than fuel. It has the power to heal.

I'll emphasize this point by citing the fact that medical researchers at the Columbia College of Physicians and Surgeons showed that more than 95% of all diseases have two fundamental or basic causes: diet and environment. This means that deficiencies of nutrients and accumulated levels of toxins contribute more to disturbed health than anything else. We need real food nutrition to build health. And the more you build health, the better your body can clean out.

Always remember: The nature of life is one of relationships. Two of them have been stressed in this little book: The relationship that exists among the many components of foods and the relationship that exists among real foods and humans. Compounds in real foods are components of an energetic matrix, a vital and intricate network that can meet the needs of your cells and their functions. It's only common sense to get your nutrition from them.

References:
Brinker, Francis, *Complex Herbs—Complete Medicines*, Sandy, OR (Eclectic Medical Publications), 2004: 73-80.
Buhner, Stephen Harrod, *The Lost Language of Plants*, White River Junction, VT (Chelsea Green Publishing), 2002: 84-85.

Burris, Ken, "These Supplements May Save Your Life...Or Not," *Eating Well*, Dec. 2006, 5 (6): 44-51.

Connolly, Declan A., "Efficacy of a Tart Cherry Juice Blend in Preventing the Symptoms of Muscle Damage," *British Journal of Sports Medicine*, Aug. 2006, 40(8): 679-683.

Cranberry-Juice Home Remedy May Really Help," *Tufts University Health & Nutrition Letter*, Apr. 2008, 26(2): 3.

DeCava, Judith A., "Let Food Be Your Medicine," *Nutrition News and Views*, Mar./Apr. 2002, 6(2): 1-6.

DeCava, Judith A. "The Lee Philosophy—Part 1," and "The Lee Philosophy—Part II," *Nutrition News and Views*, Nov./Dec. 2002, 6(6): 1-6 and Jan./Feb. 2003, 7(1): 1-6.

Doherty, James, " 'Whole Food' Supplements?," *Alternative Therapies*, Jan./Feb. 2007, 13(1): 12.

Hart, Jane, "The NIH Consensus Conference on Multivitamin/Mineral Use for Preventing Chronic Disease," *Alternative & Complementary Therapies*, Aug. 2006, 12(4): 182-186.

Howard, Brian C., " 'Pharmafoods' Feel-Good Claims: Form or Function?", *The Green Guide*, Jan./Feb. 2007, 118: 1, 4.

Low Dog, Tieraona, *Alternative and Complemetary Therapies*, Aug.2008, 14(4): 162-63.

Meletis, Chris D. and Zabriskie, Nieske, "Common Nutrient Depletions Caused by Pharmaceuticals," *Alternative & Complementary Therapies*, Feb. 2007, 13(1): 10-17.

O'Mathuna, Donal P., "Pomegranate Juice for the Prevention of Cardiac Disease and Cancer," *Alternative Therapies in Women's Health*, Dec. 2007, 9(12): 89-93.

Rogers, Sherry A., "Practicing Medicine by the Book," *Total Wellness*, Nov. 2006: 4-5.

Sarnat, Richard L., Schulick, Paul & Newmark, Thomas M., *The Life Bridge: The Way to Longevity with Probiotic Nutrients*, Brattleboro, VT (Herbal Free Press), 2002.

Savage, Geoffrey, quoted in the *New Zealand Herald*, 7 Jul. 2007.

"The Devil in the Dark Chocolate," *The Lancet*, 22/29 Dec. 2007, 370(9605): 2070.

Thomas, Tessa & Lynne McTaggart, "Are Supplements Necessary?," *What Doctors Don't Tell You*, May 2008, 19(2): 10.

"Wellness Made Easy," *UC Berkeley Wellness Letter*, Aug. 2007, 23(11): 8.

White, Linda B. "Powerful Pomegranate," *Herbs for Health*, Jun. 2008, 13(2): 31-34.

Williams, David G., "Getting the Most From Your Fruit," *Alternatives*, Feb. 2008, 12(8): 62.

Wilson, T., Singh, A.P., et al, "Human Glycemic Response and Phenolic Content of Unsweetened Cranberry Juice," *Journal of Medicinal Food*, 2008, 11: 46-54.

FOOD FOR THOUGHT

Fruits and vegetables easily lose nutrients once they are peeled or cut. The vitamin C content in some fruits can be totally lost in less than 1 hour of exposure, even in the refrigerator.

Reference: Bader, Myles H., *2001 Food Secrets Revealed*, Las Vegas NV, Northstar Publishing, 1997: 43.

The nutrient content of products you buy in the supermarket will vary so much that trying to figure out whether you are really getting what you think you are getting is just about impossible. The differences in nutritional value are caused by many factors such as storage times, transportation times, original quality of the food, washings in the markets, effects of direct light, packaging, canning procedures, freezing techniques, use of preservatives, processing, variations in the nutrient content of the soil or feed, and so on. There may be delays in getting refrigerated foods into refrigerated cases. And, sadly, some supermarkets will spray produce with chemicals to keep the fruits and veggies looking good, even though this is not supposed to happen. My garden and our farmers' market are looking better all the time.

Acerola is a fruit that resembles a cherry. It grows on a thick bush in some tropical and sub-tropical areas. It is one of—if not *the*—richest fruit sources of vitamin C complex. In 3½ ounces of the fruit there may be about 4,000 milligrams of just the ascorbic acid portion of the whole vitamin C complex.
Reference: Bader, Myles H. *2001 Food Secrets Revealed*, Las Vegas NV, Northstar Publishing, 1997: 62.

Many drugs will treat symptoms, but they cannot cure nutritional deficiencies. And nutritional deficiencies may sometimes be the reason for the symptoms in the first place.

What's a functional food? I have always considered real natural foods as functional. But these days it refers to a process wherein components of foods and nonfoods are manipulated to become "phoods"—a combination of foods and pharmaceuticals. We're talking about spiked eatables. However, the science backing these so-called functional foods is shaky. In 2003, the FDA relaxed its standards and allowed labels to tout benefits if the "weight of scientific evidence" supports a claim. This replaced the previous requirement of "significant scientific agreement" on the purported benefits. A door was opened for dubious claims. Buyer beware.

The "functional" food and drink market has already reached $19 billion in retail sales and is growing. The ads and labels promise to treat health conditions or prevent disease. Products like these really blur the lines between foods and drugs. Are they foods, or are they drugs? There's a candy strip with collagen, ceramide, and hyaluronic acid that's supposed to be good for your skin. There are baked, vitamin-fortified fruit and vegetable chips from Frito-Lay. There's the flavored water from Pepsi fortified with isolated synthetic vitamins C, E, B_3, B_5, B_6, and B_{12}. And then there's Choc-Omega, a candy that combines Belgian chocolate with omega-3 fatty acids. Such items appear to me to be nonfoods laced with chemicals. What ever happened to real food? Oh, yeah, real foods don't make as much money for manufacturers. Silly me.
Reference: "Can 'Functional Foods' Deliver on Healthy Promises?", *Tufts University Health & Nutrition Letter*, Feb. 2007, 24(12): 4-5.

You might pay more for products that have some "extra" promises-to-make-you-healthier additive, but they may provide no real added health benefits. Actually, they might even cause imbalances. Various vitamin waters are "fortified" with synthetic vitamins like A, C, E and nonfood calcium. Cereals may add soy protein. A brand of margarine boasts plant sterol and stanol esters. What we really need is a diet of real foods, not doctored foods. There are some good "functional foods" such as eggs with more omega-3 fatty acids or yogurt with probiotics. Yet these are often examples of attempts to revert back to the quality of foods which were raised Nature's way—as real foods. Hens allowed to roam free to eat insects, greens, and seeds have more omega-3s in their eggs. Properly cultured milk produces lots of probiotics, contains active cultures. Such cultured foods are best eaten fresh before the good bacteria dwindle.

Reference: Hobbs, Suzanne Havala, "What Are Phoods?", *Vegetarian Times*, Sept. 2006, 343: 28-29.

In a study from Japan, people were given supplements of dehydrated concentrates of real mixed fruit and vegetable juices. Levels of several nutrients tested showed that the supplements definitely improve nutritional status. They significantly and dramatically increased blood levels of beta-carotene, lycopene, vitamin E, and folate, for example. Levels of undesirably high homocysteine were reduced. And unhealthy breakdown of fats decreased. The scientists conducting the study concluded that fruit and vegetable juice concentrate capsules were an excellent source of nutrients that the body can use to benefit health.

Reference: Kawashima A., Madarame T., et al, "Four Week Supplementation with Mixed Fruit and Vegetable Juice Concentrates Increased Protective Serum Antioxicants and Folate and Decreased Plasma Homocysteine in Japanese Subjects," *Asia Pacific Journal of Clinical Nutrition*, 2007, 16(3): 411-421.

Researchers at the University of Florida wanted to find out if a real food supplement— in this case dried fruit and vegetable juice concentrates in capsules—would boost markers of health. They measured the blood levels of vitamin C and carotenes (beta-carotene, lycopene, and lutein) and found the supplement did indeed increase the nutrient concentrations. They also found that DNA damage was reduced and circulating amounts of certain white blood cells important to the immune system were increased. This sort of study only confirms what we have seen in real life, in clients and patients, for many years. Real food concentrates work.

Reference: Nantz, Meri P., Cheryl A. Rowe, et al, "Immunity and Antioxidant Capacity in Humans is Enhanced by Consumption of a Dried, Encapsulated Fruit and Vegetable Juice Concentrate," *Journal of Nutrition*, Oct. 2006, 136(10): 2606-2610.

Fruits and vegetables are wonderful sources of all kinds of nutrients, but they are low in enzyme content. Fresh juices, since a lot of vegetation is used, would give you more nutrients and more enzymes. Higher-calorie produce such as bananas, avocados and mangoes are actually pretty good sources of enzymes. Whole grains and meats contain more enzymes than vegetables, but when they are cooked, the enzymes are destroyed. Cooked foods cause a greater outpouring of enzymes from the body into the digestive tract than do raw foods. Cooking organically-raised meats lightly would preserve some of the precious enzymes. Properly prepared glandular supplements incorporate both the nutrient and enzyme value of these invaluable foods.

Reference: Howell, Edward, *Food Enzymes for Health & Longevity*, Twin Lakes WI, Lotus Press, 1994: 20, 26, 31, 53.

Biochemist Harold N. Simpson says that a person could spend all their time as a biochemist and "still never know all the ins and outs of all [the] various food elements." Different foods have different combinations of a myriad of elements. "So how can a person master this complex and seemingly endless list of various compounds needed for the health of the human body?" No one can master it and fabricate imitation supplements. But we can get it by eating real, natural foods and, if needed, supplements of real, natural foods. And remember, the exact needs of all the food elements are not even known. Besides, every individual is unique. Let your body choose, not a chemical-supplement manufacturer.

Reference: Simpson, Harold N., *Unhealthy Food=Unhealthy People*, Chicago, Peter Jon Simpson, Publisher, 1994: 39.

Chapter Ten

How Do I Start?

Are you feeling a little befuddled? Don't fret. Many people have the mistaken idea that eating healthy foods is too complicated, too hard, and/or too bland. It doesn't have to be any of these. Food preparation is not rocket science or brain surgery. Neither does it have to take up a big chunk of your day. It can be quite simple. From a health standpoint, it's better not to get too complicated or fancy. And eating good foods means savoring good, natural flavors. Here are five requirements to get started:

- Get really fresh, whole foods that will taste wonderful for what they are—they don't need to be hidden by myriad or exotic ingredients or multiple processes.
- You need to know how to chop and cut with a knife.
- You are able to boil water.
- You know how to turn on your oven.
- You have a desire to be a little creative, to experiment, and take small risks.

That's it. If you can do the above five things, you can prepare healthful meals.

1. *Get really fresh, whole foods.* Go to your local farmers' markets, food co-op, health food store, supermarket, meat or seafood market and get the best quality untampered-with foods you can. You may want to grow some of your own foods in your garden too—somehow the vegetables and fruit taste best when you grow them.

2. *Slice, peel, chop, grate.* Make salads, soups, stews, steamed vegetables, baked meats or poultry or seafood or vegetables or fruits. Salads are fun—they can be made with virtually any vegetable that you can eat raw, any fruit that you think you may like with them, chopped raw nuts or seeds, cheese, beans, and even bits of cooked chicken or beef or lamb if the salad is the meal. Salads can be tossed (the kind you toss and turn until all the ingredients are blended together with a dressing) or they can be composed

(kind of layered and allowed to sit as is rather than being tossed). Mix and match ingredients. Tear some greens—try various types of lettuce, cabbage, spinach, arugula, watercress, escarole, French sorrel (I love the lemony flavor), radicchio, mizuna, baby greens, whatever. Add what you found at farmers' market or what intrigues you: mild onions, bell peppers, tomatoes, celery, cucumber, radishes, any fresh herbs you like. How about grated or sliced beet root or celery root (celeriac) or fennel or kohlrabi or carrot? Toss in some parsley, fennel ferns, tender string beans, snap peas, cilantro. Sprinkle on some chopped nuts, seeds, cubes or crumbles of raw cheese, sundried olives. Slices of oranges, raisins, and other fruit go well with some salads. Dressings are easy too. About 1/3 vinegar (apple cider, wine, balsamic) or lemon or lime juice and 2/3 oil (extra-virgin olive or another unrefined type) blended together is fine with a little sea salt and freshly ground pepper. But you can be more creative than that. Bake a whole garlic bulb and squeeze out the garlic paste as a base for your dressing. Use good prepared mustard (yummy with a drizzle of raw honey and the oil of your choice), fresh salsa, real fermented soy sauce, any type of fresh herb or spice you like or that you think goes with your salad. Yogurt can be the beginning of a creamy dressing as can sesame tahini or mashed avocado. Dressings don't have to be complicated—all you need are a few ingredients, then whisk and pour. Sandwiches can start with whole grain breads to which you add whatever you imagine would taste good. This can be any number of raw veggies, raw milk cheeses, chopped nuts, seeds, spreads (such as hummus, guacamole, mashed sweet potato with grated ginger and minced onion and garlic and a little sesame oil), meat, poultry, or fish. Spreads can be made thinner with a liquid to use as dips for vegetable slices or pieces of bread.

3. *Boil water.* You can cook whole grains by soaking them several hours or overnight, then bring to a boil (just so the water begins to bubble), and turn down to low so they simmer until tender and chewy. Soft boil or poach some eggs. Scramble or fry the eggs in butter. Sauté some vegetables, then add eggs for a scramble. Brown cuts of meat or poultry in a good oil (that can deal with higher heats, like olive oil), then add cut onions, minced garlic, a liquid (water, canned or homemade broth, tomatoes with juice, or whatever you find desirable), cut or chopped veggies of choice (the ones that need the most cooking first and the ones that need the least cooking last), spices, and, finally herbs. You now have a stew or soup. You can make them with just vegetables. Or with a grain—experiment with different grains—and vegetables. Or with whole grain pasta (try brown rice pasta or whole wheat pasta). Steaming vegetables is a snap. Simply cut or slice the vegetables, put in a pot with a little bit of water, cover, bring the water to a bubble, reduce heat to low and let cook until the water is gone (you'll get the hang of how much water to use the more you do this; if the veggies aren't tender enough to eat when the water is gone, add a bit more—watch that they don't burn). Sauté some onions, garlic, mushrooms, and other vegetables; or sauté thin slices of meat, or pieces of poultry, or fish (first, try dipping in an egg wash, then cornmeal). Beans or legumes are good in soups, stews, as side dishes, in burritos or other dishes, with rice, and other ways—even salads. Soak overnight, (for small legumes like lentils or split peas, only a couple of hours are needed), discard soaking

water and replace with fresh water. Bring to a boil, turn down to a simmer, and go about your business until tender (times differ with type and size of bean). They can be added to, or you can add to them, any number of ingredients and they go with almost anything.

4. *Turn on your oven.* Meats, poultry, seafood, grains, vegetables, and some fruit (like apples) can be baked. Rule of thumb for all cooking—from a health standpoint, it is best to cook at lower rather than higher temperatures. Studies show that meats and other proteins cooked at high temperatures and carbohydrates (like grains) cooked at high temperatures produce toxins, some of which may even contribute to cancer. Interestingly, most foods you put into the oven can be baked at 350°F for 45 minutes to an hour, or at lower temperatures for longer periods of time. I have often popped some potatoes in the oven at 250° or 275° F for an hour and a half or so before eating. If you're a meat eater, cooking at low temperatures often means more tender, more juicy dishes, especially if the meat is a tougher cut. And if you want to melt some good raw milk cheese, you want the lowest possible temperature for the shortest time so you don't destroy all the enzymes or denature the protein. For baking, make sure there is some fat and often, a little bit of liquid. Fish, for instance, can be placed on a sheet of parchment paper (you can get it unbleached too) with some chopped tomato, onion, garlic, or other vegetables (which will make juice) and a pat of butter or a drizzle of oil; fold over the paper to make a packet and bake until the fish has turned from translucent to opaque. Big chunks of onion, potato, beet root, rutabaga, carrot, and other "hard" veggies are delicious baked; a light covering of oil is all they need before putting in the oven.

5. *Be creative, experiment, take small risks.* Everyone has different tastes and histories. So I can't tell you exactly what to eat or what to put into your dishes and meals. For most things, you don't need a recipe. Use what is in season, what is available; what appeals to you. Combine ingredients that "feel" right together to you. Give it a try. Add spices and herbs that you like or that seem to go with what you're making. Sometimes a dish will get raves; sometimes it will be best forgotten. Either way, you are taking risks that teach you about what works or what doesn't, what you and your family like and don't like. The best chefs in the world have created dishes that went wrong, unfortunate experiments that were thrown in the garbage or in the compost heap. Just keep in mind that if ingredient A goes with ingredient B, and ingredient C goes with B, then A will probably go as well. For example, chicken goes with onions and garlic, and pasta goes with onions and garlic, so chicken, onions, garlic, and pasta will probably make a delicious combination. Or, beans go with rice, and tomatoes go with rice, so beans, rice, and tomatoes will probably make a good base for a dish. Get some cookbooks for ideas if you want. You may need to substitute better ingredients for poorer ones listed in the cookbooks—for example, use butter instead of shortening, Rapadura (evaporated cane juice) instead of refined sugar, whole wheat flour instead of refined white flour. (Of course, some individuals should avoid all wheat products or other particular foods—whole and natural or otherwise—but this is a

matter of personal biochemistry.) Remember, cooking is an art, but baking is mostly a science and must be more precise. If you enjoy making baked items, such as bread, you will, of course, need to follow recipes, though there is often room for some small changes or additions once you get the recipes down pat.

When something you prepare turns out really good, keep in mind the things you did that worked out well or the combinations and blends that appealed to you or your family. Then you can improvise more on those things in the future. Think about what would taste good to you and, while you are preparing the dish, taste the food, look at it, smell it, and go from there. Maybe an herb or spice would be good to add, or another ingredient or two. Above all, keep it simple. Food preparation should be enjoyable, not a stress or a drag. It can be an art form, not a drudge.

Do try to eat something *raw* with each meal. Get into salads and munchies like raw vegetables, raw fruit, raw nuts and seeds, raw milk cheeses—whatever you like and can handle. (If you're not used to eating a lot of fiber that you'll get in the raw veggies and fruit, begin with small additions and gradually build up.) Don't overcook when you do cook. It's better to have most foods closer to raw than well done. If you have organic beef, for example, you don't have to cook it until it's charred and grey all the way through; leave some good pink rawness on the inside. If you steam vegetables, allow them to keep some "bite" or crispness; don't cook them into mush.

How much raw food should we eat? Opinions differ widely. Some say everything raw, others say 80% or 50%, and there are those who claim it doesn't matter. Research in the 1930s and early 1950s indicated that the human body sets off a defense reaction in the tissues of the digestive tract when cooked food is eaten. White blood cells change, there is swelling, a fever-like temperature increase, and fatigue is experienced after eating well-cooked foods. This sort of reaction also seems to take place when cooked foods are eaten first (comprising half the meal), followed by raw foods (the other half). However, when the raw foods are eaten first, this reaction doesn't take place. (Kouchakoff, Paul, [Suisse], Institute of Clinical Chemistry, Lausanne, Switzerland, "The Influence of Food Cooking on the Blood Formula of Man," Proceedings; First International Congress of Microbiology, Paris, 1930; Erasmus, Udo, *Fats that Heal, Fats that Kill,* Burnaby BC Canada, 1993: 317-318) The message is that we should have raw foods every time we eat, and, if possible, they should be the first things we eat (if we are also having cooked foods). Isn't it interesting that recent research finds that one good way for overweight folks to lose the surplus ballast is to begin each meal with a salad or with other raw foods?

One reason raw foods do not cause the defense reaction that cooked foods cause is that their enzymes help digest these foods and anything else we eat. When we eat cooked foods, our digestive glands must secrete more enzymes to accomplish the work of digestion. Fermented, enzyme-rich foods—not pasteurized for shelf life—such as homemade sauerkraut, yogurt, and others, provide plenty of friendly bacteria for intestinal health and other health benefits, plus they are easy to digest. In some cases, raw foods have a higher content of essential nutrients (for example, some vitamins are destroyed when foods are cooked). But there are limits. Raw potatoes are nutrient-dense (did you know they are an excellent source of vitamin C and protein?), but most people don't find raw potatoes tasty. Raw dried beans have a hard core and contain a protein factor that causes indigestion as well as nutrient inhibitors; but when they are germinated (soaked) and cooked, that protein factor and nutrient inhibitors are destroyed so you get more benefit from the beans. The bottom line is to eat as many raw foods as you, personally, can. And definitely begin each meal with plenty of good, raw foods.

The old adage to keep everything in moderation applies to food as well. Too much of any one thing may upset your personal biochemistry. Some individuals can eat a lot of fruit, for example, and thrive on it, whereas others don't feel as well doing so. Substituting fresh fruit for pastry and cookies is a huge improvement. But how much fruit you eat depends on what your body tells you. The same principle applies to all foods. Some variety is needed for every one of us.

Remember, *we tend to like foods we are used to eating.* Changing your diet may be one of the most difficult things you've ever done. Changing to real foods when you are used to eating mostly nonfoods may be quite a challenge.

In his book, *Eating Well,* Bart Potenza states, "They say it's harder to change people's food habits than their religion or politics."

Yes, we definitely need to motivate ourselves to change. It may not be easy, but with diligence, persistence, and plain 'ole stubbornness, it can be accomplished.

Over the years I have had oodles of people tell me that, after switching to more healthful foods for a period of time, they grew to like them more and more. If they splurged on some nonfood—such as fast food, cake at a special occasion or candy—it just didn't taste as good as they remembered. Their preferences evolved and they subsequently enjoyed the flavors and textures of real foods more than the nonfoods they used to like. However, there are some folks who never lose their desire for certain junk foods. This attachment probably comes more from their brains than their bodies—our bodies certainly want good real food over sad nonfood. Habits, memories, traditions, and associations (such as reward or comfort) are darned hard to compete with. Then there is convenience and availability: nonfoods are everywhere and often ready-to-eat. Perhaps you are simply in the habit of eating something at mid-morning or mid-afternoon and a candy bar or a couple of cookies are easily at hand. Why not try eating a piece of raw fruit, or a carrot, or some raw almonds, or something else that will not only satisfy you, but will feed your cells without adding excess weight? Or, why not try drinking a glass of good, clean water with or without your snack? Sometimes our bodies are thirsty (and most over-processed foods tend to dehydrate us anyway) more than hungry.

So remember that it's what you eat most of the time that matters. There will be special occasions when you will have a piece of cake or have that non-organic cheese in a restaurant. But to get in the good-food groove, you may need to begin slowly and gradually use more and more of the good stuff and less and less of the sad stuff. (For example, if you're used to refined white rice, begin your change by using three-quarters white rice and one quarter brown rice; next time use half white and half brown, and so on until its all brown rice.) Some diligence is needed; it's easy to slip back into old habits. Keep your goal in mind. It's like climbing up several flights of stairs after you spent many years walking down those stairs. You might begin by bounding up two steps at a time, but then you will slow down and perhaps back down a few. Don't quit! All you have to do is resume your journey upward, one step at a time. And you may come to plateaus occasionally.

Although at times you may feel that you may as well chuck it all—that this is just another diet or wellness plan that didn't work, that you should look for another health program—think again. You know the basic principles are true. All you need to do is find your way of applying them, to make this guide or strategy your own, your style. Look at how far you have come, not just how far you have to go. Do your best to move in the right direction. Focus more on what you *can* eat (the good foods you want to eat) rather on what you *can't* eat (the nonfoods you want to avoid). You know where you are going and you are learning how to get there. It's the *progress* and it's the *process*—a process of healing. You're worth it.

And, yes, real food supplements are usually more expensive than separate-chemical or fabricated-nutrient supplements. You're worth it in this area too. We are bombarded with ads and testimonials bragging about the magical advantages of taking certain high-potency synthetic vitamins or non-food minerals, or separate amino acids, or "standardized" (a high amount of a certain substance added) herbs. We are promised that other people have been cured of their diseases and had tremendous improvements in their energy, sex-lives, and appearance. "Anti-aging" is especially catchy. Folks, let's face it. We are attracted to magic and we want to believe it works.

But, the real miracles occur more quietly, gradually, deeply, and truly when we take in real, honest-to-goodness food, containing the materials Nature intended we use for our health and well-being. Your body needs to be treated with reverential respect and nurturing, compassionate understanding—this means consistently feeding it wholesome, nutrient-dense, natural real food. Step by step, the healing takes place. This is especially important to us baby-boomers who are beginning or getting close to retirement. We want to retire and live as long as possible with good health. Our day-to-day diet, our supplements, our physical activities, our outlook—all these things count.

It's just that we have been conditioned to want instant magic (remember, magic is sorcery, slight-of-hand—or shall we say "slight-of-ad"). We've been brainwashed into the "quick-fix" mentality. We seek simple, little-or-no effort solutions rather than correcting underlying systemic causes. Part of the reason we want instant magic is that we're used to the concept of drugs providing instant relief. Sometimes we do get instant reactions from synthetic supplements or junk foods. Perhaps we get a quick boost of energy or temporary suppression of a symptom. These are either shallow masking effects or efforts by our bodies to get rid of something foreign, not lasting healing or wellness. Real foods and real food supplements are not magic and they're not instant. They are, in the true sense, miraculous, wondrous, health-*full*. I can't count the number of times I have been amazed and dazzled at the incredible improvements I have seen in and heard from people who stuck with their efforts to eat well and were consistent in taking their real food supplements, along with other positive lifestyle adjustments. I've seen it over and over, but I still continue to be awed. Nature is pretty impressive.

If you are having one or more health problems, it would no doubt be best to consult a knowledgeable health professional. In this way you will get assistance for determining what the problem actually entails and what you can do about it. Sometimes medication or surgery is absolutely necessary. But very often, illnesses and unhealthy conditions can be prevented or aided by a healthy lifestyle that includes optimal nutrition. If foods and supplements will help, you can get guidance and direction regarding an individualized diet plan and specific supplements that you may need.

For example, if you have dry, scaly skin, you may need more good fats and fat-soluble vitamins such as vitamin A complex. Or you may be having difficulty in digesting fats, creating a deficit. Or you may have an underactive thyroid that results in dry skin. Or you may be experiencing a reaction to the detergent you use to wash your clothes, to your soap or other cosmetic item. Or there may be another reason.

Are you feeling especially tired? Is it a deficiency of nutrients such as the vitamin B complex, any number of minerals, protein, or essential fatty acids? If you begin the day with some energy that wanes as the day goes on, there may be adrenal gland fatigue. If it is really difficult to get out of bed but you get a little get-up-and-go later in the day, it may be an underactive thyroid. If you are a woman with heavy menstrual periods, you might be anemic. If you are a woman in your 50s, perhaps you are going through menopause. Have you been reckless with your diet, perhaps eating too many sweets and processed foods? Or have you been dieting to lose weight, maybe following the wrong diet for you or eating too little or just too little of certain nutrients you need? There are many, many reasons for fatigue.

Maybe you are concerned about the possibility of developing heart disease, or having a stroke, or getting cancer, or developing osteoporosis, or diabetes, or Alzheimer's disease, or just looking older than you should. Are there some signs or symptoms that frighten or concern you? Then find out what they may mean and what you can do to prevent many of the degenerative diseases that plague this country.

More and more people are reacting in a negative manner to the many chemical poisons and toxins that permeate our earth these days. Could some of the troubles you are experiencing be such reactions? Could you have some food intolerances that are disturbing your whole system or causing particular problems?

Are you feeling depressed, overly anxious, or are you suffering from insomnia, irritability or bursts of anger, or are you experiencing some other disorder associated with your brain? Is it just the stress you are experiencing in your life or could you be deficient in nutrients, having reactions to toxins, experiencing hormonal imbalances, or suffering with a damaged digestive system? There may be other reasons as well. You need to find out.

Do you bruise easily? Is there a bit of pink blood on your toothbrush when you brush your teeth? Do you have varicose veins or hemorrhoids? These can be signs of increased fragility of blood vessel walls which usually entails a deficiency of the vitamin C complex, especially its rutin and flavonoid components. You may also need vitamin E complex. Or there may be other contributing factors such as a lowered platelet count or something else.

If your ankles turn or you get muscle or ligament injuries frequently; if your bones break easily, or your joints pop or crack; if "oh, my achin' back" is your theme song; or if you have other musculoskeletal symptoms, you may be able to get nutritional help. Total bioactive protein, numerous minerals (not just calcium, but also magnesium, potassium, boron, manganese, and many others), vitamin C complex, and other nutrients may be needed. It could be that you need more of some than of others.

Perhaps you get colds or the flu too often. Maybe you have sinusitis at certain times of the year, or your colds tend to progress into bronchitis. Possibly you have a history of pneumonia, or asthma, or some other form of respiratory distress. It could be that your immune system needs some support, or that the tissues in the respiratory tract are not as healthy and resilient as they should be. You may be nutritionally depleted by a not-so-healthy diet or from allergies or intolerances or pollution. Find out.

Hey guys, do you have to urinate more times than you can count? It could be that you have an enlarged prostate. Or there may be some other problem. Certain foods, nutrient complexes, and herbs may be able to assist greatly.

Okay, gals, are you suffering with PMS, heavy or irregular menstrual periods, or are you having a difficult time going through menopause? Nutrition may play a role in helping out. There are nutrients necessary for proper function of your ovaries, adrenals, and other glands that produce hormones which may be imbalanced.

Do you retain fluid? Maybe you aren't getting enough fluids in your diet, or maybe you need some minerals or other nutrients to aid fluid elimination, or perhaps there is a weakness in your heart "pump" so your lower legs and feet don't get the circulation they need. Or there may be some glandular imbalance. Do you experience urinary tract inflammation or infection? It could be that the tissues lining the urinary tract need some nutritional support or that you are deficient in nutrients that allow for the proper elimination of fluids and waste, or it may be that your immune system has nutritional needs that aren't being met, or something else may be involved.

Have you tried just about every weight-loss diet devised but still can't seem to keep off the extra ballast? Perhaps you need help determining the best foods for your unique biochemistry. Or there may be a toxic condition that needs to be approached. Your liver and gallbladder might benefit from nutritional support, or there may be deficiencies of nutrients that affect your appetite and/or ability to lose weight or maintain a healthy weight.

Are you burping or belching after every meal? Do you get bloated and have too much intestinal flatulence (gas)? Maybe you suffer with heartburn or you have trouble digesting certain types of foods such as fats, fried foods, spices, or concentrated proteins such as meats and eggs, or perhaps wheat or other grains, or something else. Nutrition can help support the function of the digestive organs—your stomach, small intestine, pancreas, gallbladder. Nutrition can aid in healing a damaged or goofed-up gut. You may have food intolerances because of a leaky gut and messed up micro-creatures. Professional assistance can help you pin down your specific difficulties.

No matter what the symptom, you need to get an idea of why it's there. Symptoms are messages from our bodies. Rather than masking the symptom, we need to discover the underlying cause. We may need some assistance in determining the message, what it means, and what options we have for helping the body heal and rebalance. Ultimately, you need to take charge and follow through on what you learn to be the most beneficial course to take—for you as an individual. But having guidance and care and encouragement are usually extremely useful and advantageous.

Working into a healthful, whole-foods diet will benefit anyone and everyone. Real food supplements (with competent professional advice) will help you make up for deficiencies and imbalances you may have. What are you waiting for?

Why not get started this very day?

Suggested Reading:

Anderson, Pam, *How to Cook Without a Book*, New York, Random House Inc, 2000.
Sindell, Cheryl, *Cooking Without Recipes*, New York, Kensington Publishing Corp, 1997.
(Note: The above two books are helpful for teaching you concepts. Some ingredients mentioned may not be real foods, so substitute. Or simply absorb the principle being explained.)

Gustavs, Katharina, *Super Breakfast Cereals*, Vancouver, Canada, Alive Books, 2000.
Haas, Elson M., *A Cookbook for All Seasons*, Berkeley, CA, Celestial Arts, 2000.
LaPlace, Viana, *Unplugged Kitchen*, New York, William Morrow and Company, Inc, 1996.

Waters, Alice *Chez Panisse Café Cookbook*, New York, HarperCollins Publishers, 1999, and any of her other cookbooks.

There are innumerable cookbooks out there—some of them are very helpful in providing ideas and some of them are wonderful "natural food" cookbooks. You probably have several books already. Traditional family recipes can be adjusted, if needed, to make them healthful. There are even desserts that can be made for special occasions using more whole, natural ingredients. The truth is we really don't need more cookbooks. All we need is to master some simple, basic cooking or food preparation techniques and put together satisfying, delicious meals using the freshest whole natural foods available in our area. And we need to get in touch with our own bodies and give them what they need and want.

P.S.: If you are taking real food supplements, you will usually want to take them at the same time you eat food (unless instructed otherwise by your health professional). After all, they are food and should be part of your meals.

FOOD FOR THOUGHT

North Americans eat too many empty (de-nutritionalized) and not enough nutrient-dense foods. What influences these choices?

• *Food appeal*—primarily flavor of food, followed by appearance and personal preferences.

• *Health considerations.* Nutrition comes in second to taste in importance when selecting foods. But health appears to have little effect over the importance of convenience, except when children are present in the household.

• *Concern about weight, physical appearance, and attractiveness.* For many people, this is a more important motivator than health overall. For some reason, the visual aspect of one's body supercedes the consideration of health.

• *Money, time, and effort.* The cost of food in the US averages 10% of income, down from 14% in 1970. About 40% of each food dollar buys food prepared outside the home, up from 26% in 1970. In 1965, North Americans spent an average of 44 minutes preparing meals and 21 minutes cleaning up. By 1995, just 27 minutes included preparing meals and clean-up took four minutes. In 1987, 43% of all home-cooked meals contained at least one item made from scratch; by 1997, this rate decreased to 38%. More than 90% of North Americans consume food each day that was prepared away from home.

• *Marketing (including advertising), safety, and other factors.* In 1997, $11 billion was spent on marketing *just* fast foods.

Where are our priorities? We seriously need to consider what we are putting into our bodies. Where do we start?

Research suggests that people who have more knowledge about nutrition tend to eat

168

healthier diets than those who are less well-informed. You are already on your way because you are beginning to learn more about nutrition.

Reference: About, Jaclyn Mauer and Carol Byrd-Bredbenner, "The State of the American Diet," *Topics in Clinical Nutrition*, July-September 2007, 22(3): 202-233.

Do packaged and processed "convenience" foods really save you time? Nope. In total time—from start until plating your dinner—they won't save you even one minute, according to a study performed by UCLA researchers. They found that many families combined convenience foods with "home cooking" of raw ingredients. Those who relied most heavily on convenience foods saved only 10 to 12 minutes of hands-one preparation (such as peeling and chopping) compared to those using less packaged and processed items. But, using more convenience foods did not save any time at all in *total* meal preparation time. However (are you paying attention?) convenience foods do put a lot more refined sugar, altered fats, and additives on your plate. Prepackaged chopped or shredded raw foods lose a lot of their original nutritional content. Starting from scratch with raw foods definitely lessens ingestion of toxins and boosts your meal's nutritional value.

Reference: "Convenience Foods Don't Save Time," *Tufts University Health & Nutrition Letter*, Nov. 2007, 25(9): 3.

Let's fast-forward a few hundred years from now. Can you imagine someone writing a little book like this? It will tell of companies manufacturing a little white pill, sometimes coating it with different colors, as a "cure-all" for many ills. It was aspirin, a drug that posed serious risks like bleeding, eye disease, even heart attack and stroke. The book will relate that people actually sprayed all their farms, gardens, and orchards with poisons to kill weeds and bugs, but then the people and their meat animals ate the vegetables, fruits, and grains. In the process, they poisoned themselves. They fed their animals things that the animals wouldn't normally eat and the animals became sick. Then the people ate the meat and became sick themselves. And how amazing that the people would actually eat concoctions of industrialized materials that were not genuinely foods. Then they tried to make up for not getting what they needed by taking pills and powders made of chemicals. Why didn't they eat real food? It must have been a very strange world back then, when people were dying from heart attacks, and things called diabetes and cancer. How misguided they were.

This kind of historical account doesn't have to be. We do have a choice. All we need is the motivation and the passion to make the changes needed. Do you remember the first time you fell in love? You made changes in your life, adjustments to win your love. The changes weren't difficult to make because you were driven by the fervor, the excitement, the desire, the intense interest. Perhaps the little book of the future could be a love story instead—love of oneself, love of all life on the earth, love of the earth itself. You now have a little better understanding of the situation we are in, the choices we can make, and the consequences of the paths we can take. You can put forth the effort to make a positive transition to a healthier lifestyle. Knowledge, optimism, and love of life foster constructive action. Then the little book could end with: "And they lived healthfully ever after."

ABOUT THE AUTHOR

Judith DeCava has worked independently, as well as an associate, with physicians, nutritionists, and clinical psychologists over the past 30 years. She was chief consultant for R. Murray & Associates, Inc., of Florida and Missouri, being privileged to work with and learn from Richard P. Murray, D.C., a brilliant biochemist, doctor, humanitarian, friend and disciple of Dr. Royal Lee. After Dr. Murray's death, DeCava opened her own private practice as well as a research and consulting business in supplement formulation.

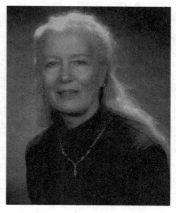

DeCava has been writing about health science since 1985 in articles, newsletters, and books. She was a regular contributor to the National Academy of Research Biochemists, Institute of Practical Biochemistry, and Biomedical Health Foundation. In her most well-known book, *The Real Truth about Vitamins and Antioxidants,* she describes the superiority of food complexes over isolated and synthetic chemical portions. She currently researches and publishes a bi-monthly newsletter, *Nutrition News and Views,* for health professionals, although it is frequently shared with the general public. (Available at IFNH's website ifnh.org)

Her interest in nutrition and health began in her teens with a search to ascertain answers to her own health problems and a fascination with the influence and effects of foods and nutrition. At first, following the dictates of current scientific and general literature on health and nutrition, the use of isolated, synthetic, and inorganic supplements were tried. After some years of working with physicians and becoming increasingly disappointed, confused, and puzzled with this line of "fake" — only barely effectual—therapy, she continued to hunt for answers, sure that there was some way, some pieces to the gigantic puzzle that would be more helpful. When, by accident, she obtained several newsletters written by Dr. Murray, the dawn began to break. A whole new world began to open with the revelation that whole foods and whole food nutritional complexes (supplements) were the factors for which people were starving, that deficiencies and imbalances were behind many ills and physical problems. Through some interesting circumstances and sheer determination, she eventually began to work with Dr. Murray and quickly became a consultant in his office for his patients. The lessons learned in practical biochemistry, anatomy, physiology, psychology, and plain old compassion went far beyond anything that could be absorbed in any of the formal courses she took or literature she read.

DeCava feels the more she learns, the more there is to learn. Her regard for Nature has always drawn her and elicited awe and reverence. Loss of health, in her view, frequently means the individual has lost touch with Nature, including loss of connection with his or her own body and Self. Rediscovering that connection with Nature and Self, including the use of Nature's foods and therapies, has become the goal of her own practice and the direction of her philosophy and writing.

Judith A. DeCava is a licensed nutrition counselor (Florida), certified dietitian-nutritionist (New York), certified nutritional consultant (organizational), professional member of the International Foundation for Nutrition and Health, American Association of Nutritional Consultants, Price-Pottenger Nutrition Foundation, American Botanical Council, associate member of the American College of Nutrition, and member of the American Association for the Advancement of Science, Weston A. Price Foundation, American Herb Association, and the National Coalition Against the Misuse of Pesticides.

INDEX

We Thank the Following Contributors of Educational Materials

John Brady, the director of IFNH, for support in compiling this manuscript into a book to help perpetuate the awareness of whole food nutrition.
International Foundation for Nutrition and Health
3963 Mission Blvd.
San Diego CA, 92109
Tel 858-488-8932
Website www.ifnh.org

Joan Grinzi, the executive director of PPNF, for granting the use of Dr. Weston Price's photos from his original study of primitive people showing the impact of what he called the "Foods of Commerce."
Price Pottenger Nutritional Foundation
7890 Broadway
Lemon Grove, CA 91945
Tel 619 462-7600
Website www.**ppnf**.org

Julia Irons, widow of V.E. Irons, who, following her husband's footsteps, graciously allowed the use of the chromatograms that dramatically show the difference between nature's vitality in whole foods versus processed foods. Dr. Royal Lee, along with V.E Irons, helped establish the National Health Federation to carry on the crusade of educating the public on the benefits of whole natural foods.
V.E. Irons and Company
P.O. Box 34710,
N Kansas City, MO 64106
Tel 816-221-3719
Website www.**veirons**.com

Recommended Educational Resources

International Foundation for Nutrition and Health
3963 Mission Blvd.
San Diego CA, 92109
Tel 858-488-8932
website www.ifnh.org/patient

IFNH was granted stewardship of the Lee Foundation for Nutritional Research, originally founded in 1943, by Dr. Royal Lee. IFNH prints and publishes many of the articles and books by Dr. Lee and other nutritional pioneers in an effort to promote the awareness and use of whole food nutrition through the practitioner.

Price Pottenger Nutritional Foundation
7890 Broadway
Lemon Grove, CA 91945
Tel 619 462-7600
Website www.ppnf.org

PPNF, originally chartered in 1952, is one of the oldest nutrition foundations in the country. It was assigned the responsibility for housing Dra.' Weston A. Price and Francis Pottenger's research on nutrition. All of the references to Dr. Weston Price's work you see today are from PPNF archives.

Recommended Reading

The following titles are available through The International Foundation for Nutrition and Health. Visit www.ifnh.org or call (858) 488-8932.

Books by the Author

The Real Truth about Vitamins & Antioxidants	ISBN 0-9645709-8-X
Vaccinations, Examining the Record	ISBN 0-9465709-7-1
Cholesterol Facts and Fantasy	ISBN 0-9645709-5-5
Nutrition News and Views: Bi-monthly newsletter	www.ifnh.org or (858) 488-8932

Additional Reading

Health vs. Disease by Dr. Melvin E. Page,	ISBN 0-9713314-4-8
Nutrition and Physical Degeneration by Dr. Weston Price	ISBN 0-87983-816-7
Food and Behavior by Barbara Reed Stitt	ISBN 0-939956-09-8
Pottenger's Cats by Dr. Francis Pottenger	ISBN 09645709-8-X
Going Back to the Basics of Human Health by Mary Frost	ISBN 978-0-9795038-0-1
Why Do I Need Whole Food Supplements? Lorrie Medford	ISBN 978- 0-9676419-3-5
New Natural Healing Cookbook by Dr. Bessie Joe Tillman	ISBN 978-0-9816238-0-1
Fats That Heal Fats That Kill by Udo Erasmus	ISBN 0-920470-38-6
Lick the Sugar Habit by Dr. Nancy Appleton	ISBN 0-89529-768-X
Empty Harvests by Dr. Bernard Jensen & Mark Anderson	ISBN 0-89529-558-X
Adrenal Fatigue by Dr. James L. Wilson	ISBN 1-890572-15-2
Dr. Bob's Guide to Stop ADHD by Dr. Robert DeMaria	ISBN 978-0-9728907-1-7
Conversations in Nutrition by Dr. Royal Lee	ISBN 0-9713314-2-1
Vitamin News by Dr. Royal Lee	ISBN 0-9713314-1-3
Dr. Royal Lee and Let's Live Magazine Articles by Dr. Royal Lee	ISBN 978-0-9840695-3-8
The Key to Better Living by Anita Shattuck